SEXOLOGY IN MIDWIFERY

Edited by **Ana Polona Mivšek**

Sexology in Midwifery
http://dx.doi.org/10.5772/57593
Edited by Ana Polona Mivšek

Contributors

Ana Polona Mivšek, Anita Jug Došler, Barbara Domajnko, Teja Zakšek, Zalka Drglin, Christian Gostečnik, Tanja Repič Slavič, Andreja Kvas, Metka Skubic, Tita Stanek Zidarič, Doroteja Rebec

Published by InTech

Janeza Trdine 9, 51000 Rijeka, Croatia

Publishing Process Manager Danijela Duric
Technical Editor InTech DTP team
Cover InTech Design team

First published April, 2015
Printed in Croatia

Additional hard copies can be obtained from orders@intechopen.com

Sexology in Midwifery, Edited by Ana Polona Mivšek
p. cm.
ISBN 978-953-51-2041-4

For EU product safety concerns:
IN TECH d.o.o., Prolaz Marije Krucifikse Kozulić 3, 51000 Rijeka, Croatia,
info@intechopen.com or visit our website at intechopen.com.

Meet the editor

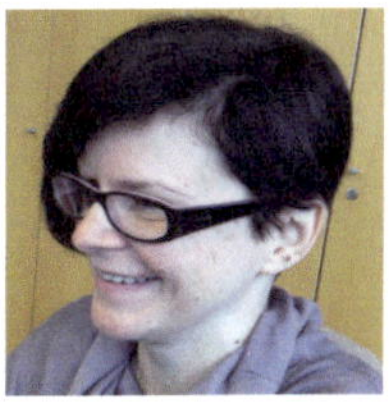

Since graduating as a first BSc midwife in 2000 (after a period of 14 years when there were no midwives trained in Slovenia) Polona Mivšek has become the first midwifery educator in Slovenia in 2002 and is currently the only midwife with a PhD in Slovenia. Currently she is Head of midwifery chair at the Faculty of Health Sciences Ljubljana. She is lecturing midwifery and since 2007 she is leading also a course of Sexology in midwifery for undergraduate midwifery students. She strongly believes that in order to manage midwifery care with empathy, midwives need to reflect upon their own points' of view (and also prejudices) regarding sexual issues.

Contents

Preface IX

Chapter 1 **Do midwives Need Sexology in Their Undergraduate Study Programme? Study Among Graduates of Midwifery Programme who Attended Sexology Course 1**
Ana Polona Mivšek

Chapter 2 **Raising Children for a Healthy Sexual Relationship in Adulthood 21**
Anita Jug Došler

Chapter 3 **Promotion and Health Education for Healthy Sexuality 33**
Andreja Kvas

Chapter 4 **Midwifery Students' Perception of Intimate Touch in Clinical Practice 67**
Tita Stanek Zidarič and Metka Skubic

Chapter 5 **Sexual Activity during Pregnancy in Childbirth and after Childbirth 87**
Teja Škodič Zakšek

Chapter 6 **The Experience of Pregnancy, Childbirth and Motherhood in Women with a History of Sexual Abuse 117**
Tanja Repič Slavič and Christian Gostečnik

Chapter 7 **Female Sexuality and Medicine – Sexualisation of Everyday Life, Desexualisation of Childbirth 143**
Zalka Drglin

Chapter 8 **Towards Unprejudiced Midwifery Care — Midwifery Students' Views on Homosexuality 165**
Barbara Domajnko

Chapter 9 **Breaking Down Taboos Concerning Sexuality among the Elderly 189**
Doroteja Rebec, Igor Karnjuš, Sabina Ličen and Katarina Babnik

Preface

Sexual health is an element of general health. It is therefore very important that health professionals are aware of the impact of individual's sexuality on clients' well-being. Together with aspects of spirituality and emotional well-being, sexuality sets the ground for the quality of life.

I claim that awareness of sexual component of human being is crucial for midwives, who deal with pregnancy, birth, puerperium, reproductive and gynaecological issues etc. These are situations that are all closely connected with intimacy, privacy and sexuality. The logical derivation is that midwives should be capable of handling the conversation and counselling on different sexual topics, setting aside their own opinions and prejudices regarding the sexuality.

The idea for the book Sexuality and midwifery arose from this point of view. There are a lot of professional circumstances we wanted to cover in the publication, but the initiative wish had to be narrowed and reduced.

All authors are academic teachers with practical experience in taking care for women. Their experiences, knowledge and expertizes provide a notable insight in the issue, with the common wish to improve the management of sexual issues within the midwifery/heath care.

The chapter written by Anita Jug Došler, PhD reviews how the consciousness regarding the sexuality in individuals develops. Andreja Kvas, PhD describes basic principles of successful health education regarding sexual matters. Metka Skubic, MSc and Tita Stanek Zidarič, MSc write about how midwives have to be empathic and aware of the women's intimate space, which they often intrude when providing a midwifery care. While Teja Škodič Zakšek, MSc describes the sexuality during normal pregnancy, childbirth and the postnatal period, Tanja Repič, PhD deals with these periods of life through the ocular of the woman who was abused in the past. Zalka Drglin, PhD using feminist approach, discusses female sexuality in relation to modern medicine. Barbara Domajnko, Phd describes a research regarding midwifery students' views on homosexuality and a team of researchers - Doroteja Rebec, MSc, Igor Karnjuš, MSc, Sabina Ličen, MSc and Katarina Babnik, PhD presents the data of the study regarding the sexuality among elderly.

All above issues are a part of the curriculum of the subject Sexology in midwifery that I lecture to the undergraduate midwifery students, attending BSc midwifery programme at the Faculty of health sciences Ljubljana. The experiment started with the programme accredited in 2004. The evaluation of the subject after providing these contents to the midwifery students for 10 years shows that midwifery students do think that discussion about sexual issues have to be a part of the formal education. They estimated the subject as helpful and important.

I hope that with drawling their attention to these topics, I contribute to the future generations of empathic and sympathetic midwives, who will practice woman-centred care, focusing on all aspects of her well-being.

Ana Polona Mivšek
Head of the Department of Obstetrics / Department of Midwifery
University of Ljubljana, Slovenia

Chapter 1

Do midwives Need Sexology in Their Undergraduate Study Programme? Study Among Graduates of Midwifery Programme who Attended Sexology Course

Ana Polona Mivšek

Additional information is available at the end of the chapter

http://dx.doi.org/10.5772/59007

1. Introduction

The midwife is recognized worldwide as being the person who is alongside and supporting women giving birth. The midwife also has a key role in promoting health and well-being of childbearing women and their families before conception, antenataly and postnataly, including family planning [1]. The role expands to the field of family planning and promoting sexual health [2]. Since midwives work on the field of perinatal health, but also in the field of gynaecology and reproduction, they face different situations that are closely connected with sexuality.

Despite the fact that our societies become much more open and relaxed regarding the sexual issues, there are still hindrances to discuss the issue freely with someone you are not familiar with [3,4]. So women do need trust in midwives, before they open to reveal the concerns, problems or hesitations on the topic. And midwives should be educated in how to manage delicate situations, concerning sexual problems. Definition of Midwives acknowledge midwives' role in managing sexuality [5] and International Confederation of Midwives request this competency to be met within the undergraduate education [6], but on the other side, midwifery textbooks are very parsimonious on this topic [1,7].

In order to equip the Slovenian midwifery students with knowledge and skills about managing sexuality issues, the subject Sexology in midwifery was introduced into the undergraduate midwifery programme in 2004. It ran continuously every year until today. This chapter presents the results of the evaluation of the subject, by the graduates of midwifery, who attended the course.

2. Background

The focus that this chapter deals with, lays in the cross-section of midwifery and sexuality, however these two components is hard to separate completely. The state of the motherhood is obviously bound up with definitions of sexuality. The interlinking with sexual identity, sexual activity and motherhood is very complex tangle to unpick [8]. Midwifery is closely connected with sexuality of a couple; the birth is the take of the period that started with the sexual act. As sexual intercourse is not just the physical act, also pregnancy, birth and processes after the birth cannot be considered only bodily – they are multidimensional in its nature, affecting emotions, social and spiritual aspects of individual. These effects are not limited only to woman, but affect the family as a whole.

The intercourse, pregnancy, childbirth, breastfeeding and establishment of new relationships after the birth are very intimate milestones of the family life. As Price [9] acknowledges: "The physical changes of woman are linked also to her views of her sexual self". Her changing physical shape reveals that she is recognized by others as a sexual being [10].This process affects all aspects of her life.

The midwife that actively enters in the life of the couple/family during these periods must be therefore consciously aware of the emotional value of these periods for the clients. Already in 1975 World Health Organization acknowledged [11]: "Opportunities for the provision of sex information and counselling are particularly likely to arise in services for maternal and child health, family planning, mental health, community health, abortion and sterilization, and sexually transmitted diseases".

2.1. Midwifery

There are many subthemes of midwifery that are closely connected to the management of issues of sexuality, however because of the above reasons, the author exposed the most evident connections, such as empathy or emotional work, communication skills and ethics.

2.1.1. Empathy and emotional work

Empathy is essential for the effective provision of midwifery care [12]. However, in case of dealing with sexuality issues, is even more crucial. It helps midwife not to invade in womens' intimacy. In relating empathy to the therapeutic relationship of a midwife, it is seen to require midwife to be intuitive, with the woman then being able to show the depth of her understanding of another person [13].

It was Hochschild who was the first person exposing the importance of emotions in work, however, his work was largely focused on commercial organizations. Emotional work in midwifery is of great importance, however largely unrecognized. Midwives need to work in a sensitive way in order that woman's feelings are acknowledged and responded to. To do this effectively, midwives also need to be aware of their own feelings, as their unrevealed inside conflicts can affect communication and relationship with women [14].

Students learn the emotional work during the study. The senior staff at the clinical placements are usually the role models for them and the perception changes over the educational process [15]. When dealing with problems in sexual area, it is of crucial meaning that midwives learn how to communicate and manage the feelings.

On the surface it could be presumed that midwifery is "on the happy side" of healthcare, and that only positive emotions will usually be felt [14]. But it is not always so. Midwives work also with clients that experience undesired pregnancy, live in an abusive relationship, have problems with conception, decide to end pregnancy etc. In these cases midwives need to support women even with greater emotional awareness.

The word partnership is often used to describe woman-midwife relationship. Some authors even go further and name it "professional friendship" [16]. Relationship between woman and a midwife can vary in its intensity, trust, openness and level of intimacy. This often depends on the level of reciprocity [17] and is closely connected with the way of communicating with each other.

2.1.2. Ethics and mode of communication

The midwife-women relationship is the foundation of the midwifery services says Kirkham [18]. The social context of those involved – their values and believes affect what the two parties bring to their relationship [19]. It is important of being aware of these sometimes unconscious impacts (or even biases), when communicating and acting.

Questions regarding sexuality may be regarded as problematic as they are sensitive and complex, and demand time and expertise [20]. In the study by Wendt et al. [21] health professionals (midwives and doctors) exposed, beside lack of organisational support or communication skills, difficult emotions that complicate the situation when speaking of sexual problems. This reason might restrain midwives and clinicians from raising sexual issues. It is important that woman is treated as a partner in a relationship, so that the solutions to her problems derive from her alone. Therefore active listening is used when discussing things with women [22].

As language, also actions, when dealing with delicate situations, which those connected to sexuality certainly are, must be tactful, sensitive and ethically sound. Attending women in childbirth is highly intimate and some procedures are very intrusive (for example vaginal examinations); midwives need to perform them with sensitivity and empathy. Especially when dealing with delicate sexuality issues (such as pregnancy after sexual abuse or similar), midwives must bear in mind that their actions and words affect women deeply.

Being ethically aware is a necessary step towards being an autonomous practitioner [23]. Believes and values of professionals and clients that interact are very different and derive from their broader social context, culture and past experiences. Therefore the solutions to same problems may vary, but there need to be clear ethical boundaries that must not be crossed.

2.2. Sexology

Sexology defined by Oxford dictionary [24], is "the study of human sexual life or relationships". On the Kinsey Institute website [25] sexology is defined in much more detail: "Sexology is the systematic study of human sexuality. It encompasses all aspects of sexuality, including attempting to characterise 'normal sexuality' and its variants, including paraphilias. Modern sexology is a multidisciplinary field which uses the techniques of fields including biology, medicine, psychology, statistics, epidemiology, pedagogics, sociology, anthropology, and sometimes criminology to bear on its subject. It studies human sexual development and the development of sexual relationships as well as the mechanics of sexual intercourse and sexual malfunction. It also documents the sexuality of special groups, such as handicapped, children, and elderly, and studies sexual pathologies such as sex addiction and child sexual abuse. Sexology is considered descriptive, not prescriptive: it attempts to document reality, not to prescribe what behaviour is suitable, ethical, or moral. Sexology has often been the subject of controversy between supporters of sexology, those who believe that sexology pries into matters held sacrosanct, and those who philosophically object to its claims of objectivity and empiricism".

The concept of sexology as a science in Europe was first proposed in 1907 by the Berlin dermatologist Iwan Bloch. His ideas were quickly embraced by interested colleagues in the same city, especially Magnus Hirschfeld, who in 1908 edited the Journal of Sexology, in 1913 co-founded the Medical Society for Sexology and Eugenics, in 1919 the Institute for Sexology in Berlin and organized the first international conference on sexology in 1921 in Berlin. Both Bloch and Hirschfeld believed that the traditional medical approach to sexual questions was too narrow and had to be broadened. Only a combination of methods taken from the natural and social sciences could do justice to the complex bio-psycho-social phenomenon of human sexual behavior [26]. The very important document that set the scene of sexology in the area of health was WHO document introduced in 1975 [11].

2.2.1. Sexual health and midwifery

It took several ages until the claim that all health professionals should have some basic scientific knowledge about human sex behaviour. It derived from the document on definition and promotion of sexual health by the World Health Organization [11]. That is to say, physicians and psychotherapists, nurses, hospital administrators, marriage and family counsellors, family planning officials, community health workers and even epidemiologists should receive at least some sexological training. But this enterprise is still marginalized in universities [26]. There is also an obvious shortage of interested teachers who can devote the necessary time to acquiring sufficient knowledge and skill in dealing with human sexuality to organize and lead educational programmes in this area [11].

Sexuality is essential to health and contributes to quality of life, personal development and well-being. Positive sexual experiences promote health when they generate a feeling of security [27]. Nursing and midwifery council [2] sees the role of the midwife in individual counselling, solving the sexual problems like advising women regarding the contraception (also appropriate for woman that breastfeeds), dealing with loss of libido (for example in the postpartum), giving advice regarding sexuality during pregnancy, solving the problems with discomfort of the perineum after the birth or even dyspareunia, dealing with problems of changed body image during pregnancy etc. One aspect of the midwifery care can be also advising about natural methods of family planning [28].

When women attend health-care services, there are opportunities to create a dialogue aimed at promoting their sexual health [29]. But often health professionals believe that they have insufficient education, feel poorly prepared and therefore they do not discuss sexual issues with their patients [30]. However women expect them to – in a study by Wendt et al. [31], a majority of young women approved of being asked about sexuality by midwife or clinician, because they trusted them [21]. Sexology training programs, whether academic or professional, must therefore be included in the basic study of health professionals, to improve attitudes as well as to impart knowledge [26].

Despite very clear role of the midwife in dealing with sexual issues, midwifery textbooks usually present only certain aspects of sexuality, such as contraception or intimacy during pregnancy and childbirth [28, 32]. The question is, where midwifery students learn the skills and approaches to address the issue of sexual health. Health-profession students commonly state that conversation about sexuality with patients makes them uncomfortable [33]. The author identified that this field of midwifery is largely neglected, however very important for women, therefore she decided to include the subject of Sexology into the undergraduate study programme of midwifery.

2.3. Midwifery study programme and sexology

In 2004 midwifery education in Slovenia faced great changes. With Slovenia entering EU, changes of curriculum had to be made to address all midwives' competencies, according to the European directives [34]. Within the implementation of the undergraduate study programme that is delivered at the Faculty of Health sciences in Ljubljana (the only midwifery programme in Slovenia), also new subject was added to the curriculum, called Sexology in midwifery. It was composed of 20 hours of lectures and was allocated in the last (third year) of the midwifery study. It was a compulsory subject [35].

With the changes of the programme in 2007, due to the Bologna reform, subject Sexology in midwifery expanded to 15 hours of lectures and 30 hours of seminars. It was still allocated in the last (third) year of the programme, however it was not mandatory anymore [36].

The content and the aim of the subject stayed the same; however the expansion enabled to discuss the themes more in depth and the use of different forms of study provided the possibility to use other teaching methods, not just lecturing.

The contents of the study are:

- views on sexuality throughout the history;
- views on sexuality in different cultures and effect of the religion on the perception of culturally acceptable sexual behaviours;

- perceptions of sexuality in postmodern society;
- individual aspects and prejudices regarding sexual issues;
- sexuality in art;
- midwives role, approach and communication regarding sexual issues;
- interconnections among love, sexuality, partnership, parenthood;
- sexuality in different periods of woman's life;
- sexuality during pregnancy, birth and puerperium;
- women's sexual problems and midwifery care [36].

The goal of the subject is that students get an insight into own standpoints and attitudes regarding certain sexual issues and through the discussion identify own barriers, prejudices and hindrances for open communication about this matter with women.

At first the only method used was lecture, but later it become evident that students appreciate also debate, projects and benefit from role playing. At first the subject had an exam at the end of the course. But since the main aim of the subject was never testing theoretical knowledge of the students, the subject is now assessed on the basis of students' work within the project/ seminar and involvement in the discussion.

Since undergraduate study programme of midwifery is going to be implemented again in 2015, there was a need to evaluate the subject in order to decide, whether to still include it into the future 4-year curriculum.

3. Methodology and research design

With the aim of evaluating the form, content, methods and employability of knowledge and skills gained through the realization of the subject Sexology in Midwifery, which is included in the undergraduate midwifery study programme, the quantitative research method was used. For the administration of the questionnaire, author used web survey, using EnKlikAnketa [37], the tool that provides the option of transmission of the data into the SPSS programme.

3.1. Research tool

The research tool was questionnaire, developed especially for the study that evaluated all aspects of the curriculum. Questionnaire was not pilot tested, however it was discussed over with methodologist and was given to two academic colleagues to fulfil and define vague questions.

Questionnaire was composed of 16 questions: 11 closed questions, 3 semi-closed questions (with the possibility "other") and 2 open ended questions. The first two questions ("Did you study midwifery" and "Did you attend subject Sexology in midwifery") were selective – if participants answered them no, they were not able to answer all the other questions. In questions regarding the general satisfaction with the subject, satisfaction with contents and teaching methods, author used Likert scale. Participants had to answer all the questions, otherwise they were not allowed to move to the next question in the survey.

3.2. Participants, sampling

The approach was total population sampling [38] - the sample included all generations of graduates of midwifery study programme, from the year, when Sexology was introduced in the study programme, till June 2014. It consisted of 174 participants. 3 mails returned with the notification that e-mail address is not active anymore, so final number of participants included in the study was 171.

3.3. Data collection, ethical considerations and analysis

Participants were approached through the alumni club list; the request with the link to the web survey was sent to them via e-mail address. The web survey was available online from 19th of June, till 20th of July 2014.

When graduates were approached, they were ensured confidentiality. It was stressed for several times (in the mail and in the introduction letter of the survey) that their cooperation is voluntary. In order to ensure participants confidentiality, we did not ask about the gender (since only few graduates in midwifery are males and would feel exposed) and the year of attendance in the subject, so it is impossible to track participants from their answers.

Data from the survey were analysed with SPSS (version 20) programme. Basic descriptive statistic measures were calculated for this paper, to get the general insight into the participants' views on the subject. Some of the results of the study are presented below.

4. Results

112 graduates participated in the survey, 26 of them did not finish the whole questionnaire, however their answers were used, where given. That gave the survey the response rate of 65%.

The majority of the participants were satisfied with the subject, as shown in Table 1.

Were you satisfied with the subject? (N=105)			
I was not satisfied at all	I was not satisfied	I was satisfied	I was very satisfied
0 (0%)	8 (8%)	58 (55%)	39 (37%)

Table 1. General satisfaction of students with the subject Sexology in midwifery

The next complex of questions evaluated the organization and the form of the subject. The first question referred to appropriateness of that the subject is in the last year of the study. Again, the majority of the participants supported the inclusion of the subject in the last year of study, but some of them (one fifth) objected. The results are shown in Table 2.

Do you think subject should be in the last year of midwifery education? (N=104)		
	N	**%**
Yes	84	81%
No	20	19%

Table 2. Participants' view regarding the instalment of the subject into the midwifery curriculum

Author asked students whether they think subject is comprehensive enough. One third of students thought it is not correctly emphasized, however the proportions of those who thought that it is too extensive and those who thought it is undervalued were evenly distributed (Table 3).

Do you think subject is correctly evaluated (3 ECTS = 90 hours of student's work)? (N=101)		
	N	**%**
Yes	72	71%
No, I would wish more hours	17	17%
No, I would wish less hours	11	11%
I do not know	1	1%

Table 3. Participants' estimation of the appropriateness of students' workload to the subject

Participants were also asked whether they think the subject should be mandatory for the midwifery students. The opinions of the participants were almost equally distributed as shown in Table 4.

Do you think the subject should be mandatory? (N=101)		
	N	**%**
Yes	59	58%
No	42	42%

Table 4. Participants' view about the mandatorily attendance of the subject

When discussing the size of the group, appropriate for the realization of the subject, half of the participants thought that the group of 30-35 students is too large. None of them thought it is too small, as shown in Table 5.

The group is very coherent, since all participants are midwifery students of the same generation and they know each other very well; they are relaxed in the company of one another and do not feel restrain to express own thoughts. If conversation turns to intimate questions it is very important that participants feel reassured that nothing will be revealed outside the group.

What do you think about the size of the group (30-35 students)? (N=101)		
	N	%
Too large	50	50%
Too small	0	0%
Just right	51	50%

Table 5. Participants' opinion regarding the size of the subject's group

Since there is an interest for the subject also from other health professions (such as nursing students, occupational therapists etc.), author asked students whether they would agree for other students to join the class. More than half of the participants disagreed (Table 6). From the open ended comments, two major themes for disagreement emerged – one revealed participants' opinion that dealing with sexual issues is not relevant for other health professionals so much as for midwives; the other important issue expressed was that other (unknown) students would affect the openness and relaxedness of discussion within the group. Since there is also a tendency to open the subject for incoming students from other countries that come to the faculty via international exchange, the participants were also asked whether they would attend the subject if run in English language. 62% of students would join the subject even if lectured in foreign language.

Should other students join the subject? (N=97)		
	N	%
Yes	46	47%
No	51	53%

Table 6. Participant's opinion about the appropriateness of multi-disciplinarity of the subject

The question that seemed even more important than general satisfaction with the subject was whether the gained knowledge seemed useful to participants for their clinical work. Only 11% of participants did not perceive information helpful, as seen in Table 7. In the open-ended section, the most often exposed general comment of these participants was that they already knew things that were discussed/lectured about and therefore they did not see the benefits.

Do you think knowledge gained was useful for midwifery practice? (N=94)		
	N	%
Gained information were helpful for my midwifery work	63	67%
Gained information were not helpful for midwifery work	10	11%
Otherwise:	21	22%

Table 7. Participants' opinion regarding the usefulness oft he gained knowledge for their clinical work

When asking participants regarding the satisfaction with the specific content of the subject, it was obvious that majority of the participants were satisfied with all included contents; the satisfaction ranged from 69% to 89%, depending on the theme. Students evaluated as best the lecture about "sexuality through history", while the content "sexuality in art" was least appreciated. More details on the evaluation of the content of the subject can be seen from the Table 8.

Were you satisfied with the content of the subject? (N=90)					
	I was not satisfied et all	I was not satisfied	I was satisfied	I was very satisfied	I was not satisfied et all
Sexuality through history	0 (0%)	7 (8%)	52 (58%)	28 (31%)	3 (3%)
Sexuality in different cultures and effect of the religion	1 (1%)	14 (16%)	34 (38%)	39 (43%)	2 (2%)
Sexuality in the postmodernism	2 (2%)	6 (7%)	32 (36%)	44 (49%)	6 (7%)
Sexuality in art	4 (4%)	14 (16%)	43 (48%)	26 (29%)	3 (3%)
Individual aspects and prejudices regarding sexual issues	0 (0%)	6 (7%)	34 (38%)	43 (48%)	7 (8%)
Approach and communication regarding sexual issues	0 (0%)	4 (4%)	32 (36%)	46 (51%)	8 (9%)
Midwives role in management of the sexual issues	1 (1%)	9 (10%)	24 (27%)	47 (52%)	9 (10%)
Interconnections among love, sexuality, partnership, parenthood	0 (0%)	6 (7%)	27 (30%)	48 (53%)	9 (10%)
Sexuality in different periods of woman's life	1 (1%)	9 (10%)	27 (30%)	46 (51%)	7 (8%)
Sexuality during pregnancy, birth and puerperium;	1 (1%)	11 (12%)	27 (30%)	45 (50%)	6 (7%)
Women's sexual problems and midwifery care	1 (1%)	8 (9%)	26 (29%)	47 (53%)	7 (8%)

Table 8. Participants' satisfaction with the content of the subject

Only few participants gave concrete answers on the open comment, where they were asked what else they think should be added as a content in the subject. Some of them proposed themes such as: sexuality of disabled people, more about the relaxed conversation with couples regarding the sexual issues. Some did not see the relevance of lectures like "sexuality through history" or "sexuality in art"; this didn't seem relevant to them for their professional work. On the other side, some of the participants would like the listed themes to be debated in much more details.

Author asked participants also how they liked different approaches to teaching that were used. The evaluation of the study methods by participants is presented in Table 9. The most negative response was to seminar work and they liked debates the most. The majority (90%) were satisfied with lectures. It might be concluded from the results that they prefer conventional teaching methods.

How were you satisfied with the teaching methods used in the subject? (N=89)					
	I was not satisfied et all	I was not satisfied	I was satisfied	I was very satisfied	I was not satisfied et all
Lectures	0 (0%)	7 (8%)	43 (48%)	37 (42%)	2 (2%)
Role playing	0 (0%)	11 (12%)	33 (37%)	30 (34%)	15 (17%)
Debates	0 (0%)	3 (3%)	28 (31%)	53 (60%)	5 (6%)
Project work	2 (2%)	6 (7%)	40 (45%)	25 (28%)	16 (18%)
Seminars	4 (4%)	12 (13%)	35 (39%)	30 (34%)	8 (9%)
Fieldwork	5 (6%)	7 (8%)	17 (19%)	16 (18%)	44 (49%)

Table 9. Participants' satisfaction with teaching methods of the subject

Next question asked participants, which method do they think would be the most appropriate to teach and learn about sexuality. Their responses are presented in Table 10 – again it was confirmed that they would like more debates and guided conversations on the topics. In the category other, they exposed also field work. Again it is very clear that they do not estimate seminar work as useful in gaining knowledge on the topic.

Which teaching method would you prefer to be used in learning about sexuality? (N=89)		
	N	%
Lectures	8	9%
Role playing	8	9%
Debates	57	64%
Project work	1	1%
Seminars	0	0%
Fieldwork	7	8%
Other	8	9%

Table 10. Preferable teaching methods of the participants for learning about sexuality

Since the aim of the subject is that participant gets the insight into their own attitudes and believes and that they relax in conversation about the delicate theme such as sexuality, the author questioned whether the exam is needed at the end of the subject. However, as presented in Table 11, only 12% of participants thought the subject should not be marked. The majority thought that the most appropriate would be to mark the exercises and home works they were assigned to.

Which type of the evaluation do you think is appropriate for this subject? (N=89)		
	N	**%**
Written exam	11	12%
Oral exam	12	13%
Mark of the exercise (seminar, project etc.)	33	37%
Collaboration in the debate	12	13%
Subject should not be marked	11	12%
Other	10	11%

Table 11. Participant s' opinions about the most appropriate examination at the end of the subject

In the category other, where students had an opportunity to explain their selection, the majority of propositions contained the idea of combining the above mentioned methods of evaluation. The most common combination was the mark of the assignments and the consideration of student involvement in the debates.

5. Discussion and conclusions

Midwifery is, as shown in the literature, closely connected to sexuality. Midwives should be those in the relationship that give woman permission and stimulation to raise also questions regarding the topic. In order to promote women's sexual health, there is a need for improved dialogue between patients and health professionals; midwives and clinicians have the main responsibility to initiate this dialogue. Communication between patients and professionals is an important part of health care [21]. Women, however, seldom raise questions regarding sexual problems [39]. And as seen from the literature, midwives and clinicians might fail to raise questions due to a series of obstacles [20].

Wendt et al. [21]. claim that one of the problems can be also that only a minority of clinicians, midwives and nurses have vocational training in sexology, and suggest that increased knowledge, support and opportunities for reflection concerning dialogue regarding sexual issues might evoke the interest and intent of health professionals to approach these issues. Authors [40], albeit considering other aspects of midwifery care connected with sexuality, suggest that critical thinking around the cultural and moral dimensions of sexuality should be emphasised in undergraduate training and continuing education, to help nurse-midwives and other health practitioners to deal more empathetically with the sexual matters.

The described subject "Sexology in midwifery" that was included in the undergraduate study programme of midwifery, aimed that midwifery graduates would understand the connection between sexuality and midwifery. However, the goal was not only to raise the awareness, but also to reflect upon students' individual perceptions and attitudes. When woman experiences problems in sexuality it is of great importance that midwife is capable to act as an emphatic professional. And there is a close relationship between attitude and behaviour [41]. Therefore it is important that student midwives are aware of their own beliefs and how these attitudes affect their professional acting and judgement.

WHO [11] identified three necessary stages in educating health professionals regarding the sexuality:

- in order to develop a better understanding of problems of human sexuality, it is necessary for health workers to develop healthy attitudes to sexuality, marriage, and contraception. An understanding by the worker of his/her own sexuality and a rational approach to his/her own sexual problems will help him/her to be better able to deal with the problems of others;

- in order to approach the topic with confidence, the health workers must themselves have accurate scientific knowledge regarding the facts of human reproduction and human sexuality; they must know what are the common sexual problems and how to deal with them;

- to enhance his or her ability to help those people who ask for help in the solving the problems related to sexuality, it is essential for the health worker to develop the necessary skills in the art of communication and good listening.

The contents of the teaching about the sexuality can be extracted from the above WHO's suggestion. WHO [11] document also warns that "where sexology is a part of the health study programme, emphasis is frequently on deviancy and pathology rather than on normal sexual development and behaviour". It can be claimed that normal sexuality is satisfactory covered in the midwifery curriculum. It is also obvious that the contents of the subject "Sexology in midwifery" are not prone to pathological sexual behaviour. The contents also do not deal only with the topics, relevant to manage sexual issues in perinatal period, but are more spread in order to give graduates the broader insight. Some of the participants did not see the relevance of certain contents, however attitudes and believes can be changed also with the subtle impressions that sometimes are not directly connected [42].

Already in the document of WHO was acknowledged that different methods in teaching about sexuality can be used to attain the best outcome: "in the more developed programmes there is a considerable amount of methodological experimentation and innovation; among the methods being tried are: panel discussions, male-female teaching teams, videotape case presentations, guest speakers from the community, and survey questionnaires for assessment of sexual attitudes and knowledge. A number of teaching methods have been selected because they oblige students to confront their own attitudes, values, and feelings regarding sexuality. Examples of these are the use of frank sexual films followed by small group discussions; interviews with homosexuals; role playing; and other methods requiring the active involvement of the learner" [11]. Especially meaningful are the methods, which enhance student's active involvement, like debates and role playing. That was identified as beneficial also from the opinions of participants in the study presented. However the debate must be grounded on the solid theoretical base that defines the theme. In order to achieve that, author often used combination of lectures and discussion.

Some of the methods, suggested by WHO [11] are in details described by Haeberle [26]: "in the USA they provide special programme for health professionals to enlighten them with different sex behaviours and prepare them to work confident but still with sensitivity with different sort of patients". These approaches certainly provide experience that leave a strong impact on the students' minds; however some of the described methods would be impossible to use in Slovenia, due to different cultural context, and lack of options. Nevertheless, both references give very clear idea that the main goal of this education is not only to teach health practitioner the approaches to discuss sexual health with clients, but aim at affecting participants' believes and prejudices. Similar than in foreign studies [43], it was exposed also by Slovenian participants that they would want more practice-based educational methods. Foreign authors acknowledge that this is hard to provide, because of the ethical barriers [43] and therefore suggest a model, where theoretical knowledge is reinforced practically with practice based scenarios and mentor emulation as staging points, which help to develop confident practice. Other authors [44, 45]. agree that problem-based scenarios can successfully replace lack of concrete situations and stimulate critical thinking.

The subject "Sexology in midwifery", taught in the undergraduate midwifery programme was overall good accepted by the students and almost all the graduates were satisfied with it. It seems that majority support the decision to put the subject in the last year of midwifery study; students are more mature, they already gain clinical experience and are well theoretically versed into the midwifery matters. Results confirmed the authors' anticipation that participants feel more relaxed in a homogenous group of midwifery students; many expressed restrains to be a part of the group of different unknown students.

Overall it seemed that subject covers the contents they expected (they did not give a lot of new suggestions to be included), however it could be improved via different and more various teaching methods. The very obvious message that derived from the results was the fact that participants would like more discussions. In parallel with this goes also their suggestion of dividing students into smaller groups. WHO [11] allows that human sexuality is taught as a required or an elective component of education. What is important is that the course organizers develop programmes that are appropriate, in both curriculum content and educational method, to sociocultural factors, the needs of students, and the health needs of the local population. It seems that the decision to alter the subject from mandatory to selective in 2007 was justified, since not all the participants are prepared to attend it and not all see the benefits of the contents for their clinical expertise, as proven from the participants' answers.

http://dx.doi.org/10.5772/59007

The dilemma regarding the evaluation in the subject still remains; author is aware that the theoretical exam undervalues the real aim of the subject, since the goal is to affect individual's thoughts. The final examination is however always a teacher's judgement of value [46]. Estimation of student's input in the case of revealing personal and intimate experiences, thoughts and perceptions can be also a matter of ethical question; the students might feel that a bad mark is a reflection of their unconventional opinions and expressed negative thoughts during the study. Therefore the authors' opinion is veering in the way of not marking the subject at all, however it seems that participants do not perceive that kind of hindrances as author.

The presented study has its limitations. For the in-depth information qualitative approach would be more appropriate, however for the first step of the study of evaluation of the subject, only a general overview was sought. The author is aware of the web-survey limitations [47, 48], but this approach also has major advantages – it is more economical, time effective and since it is adjusted to the population that was researched (students frequently use technical equipment) can improve response rate [49]. The main limitation of the research tool was that participants had to answer all the questions otherwise they were not allowed to move to the next question, which resulted in the loss of participant when progressing through the questionnaire. Still the study provides useful information how to improve the subject and gives the author the confirmation that these topics are relevant to midwives and that the general form of the subject is solid and fair.

Author details

Ana Polona Mivšek*

Address all correspondence to: polona.mivsek@zf.uni-lj.si

Faculty of health Ljubljana, Slovenia

References

[1] Fraser DM, Cooper MA (2009). The midwife. In: Myles textbook for midwives. 15th ed. Edinburgh: Churchill Livingstone, Elsevier; 3-10.

[2] Nursing and midwifery council (2004). Midwives rules and standards. London: NMC.

[3] Andolsek-Jeras L, Pinter B, Kozuh-Novak M, Obersnel Kveder D (1992). Fertility survey in Slovenia in 1989. Second Congress of the European Society of Contraception, 6-9 May 1992. Athens: ESC, 103.

[4] Jug Došler A, Mivšek AP, Korošec M (2013). Pojmovanje in doživljanje menstruacije pri študentkah babištva. Obzornik zdravstvene nege 47(1): 47-55.

[5] ICM (2011). The definition of a midwife. Avalable at: http://www.internationalmidwives.org/assets/uploads/documents/Definition%20of%20the%20Midwife%20-%202011.pdf (22.7.2014)

[6] ICM (2013). Concordance of midwifery curriculum with ICM Essential Competencies for basic midwifery practice. Available at: http://www.internationalmidwives.org/assets/uploads/documents/CoreDocuments/ICM%20Curriculum%20concordance%20map%20-revised%202013.pdf (22.7.2014)

[7] Pairman S, Pincombe J, Thorogood C, Tracy S, eds (2006). Midwifery: preparation for practice. Sydney: Churchill Livingstone Elsevier.

[8] Symonds A, Hunt SC (1996). The midwife and society: perspectives, policies and practice. New York:Palgrave Macmillan.

[9] Price J (1988). Motherhood: what it does to your mind. London: Pandora, 31.

[10] Mullin A (2002). Pregnant bodies, pregnant minds. Feminist theory 3(1): 27-44.

[11] WHO (1975). Education and treatment in human sexuality: the training of health professionals. Available at: http://www.sexarchive.info/GESUND/ARCHIV/WHOR.HTM (24.7.2014)

[12] Hall J (2001). Midwifery, mind and spirit.: emerging issues of care. Oxford: Books for midwives.

[13] Siddiqui J (1999). The therapeutic relationship in midwifery. British journal of midwifery 7(2): 111-14.

[14] Hunter B (2009). The emotional context of midwifery. In: Fraser DM, Cooper MA, eds. Myles textbook for midwives. 15th ed. Edinburgh: Churchill Livingstone, Elsevier; 11-20.

[15] Hunt S, Symonds S (1995). The social meaning of midwifery. Basingstoke: MacMillan.

[16] Pairman S (2000). Women-centered midwifery: partnerships or professional friendships? In: Kirkham M, ed. The midwife-mother relationship. Basingstoke: MacMillan; 207-225.

[17] Fleming V (1998). Women and midwives in partnership: a problematic relationship? JAN 27: 8-14.

[18] Kirkham M (2010). The maternity services context. In: The midwife-mother relationship. 2nd ed. New York: Palgrave Macmillan.

[19] Anderson L, Pelvin B (2006). Ethical frameworks for practice. In: Pairman S, Pincombe J, Thorogood C, Tracy S, eds (2006). Midwifery: preparation for practice. Sydney: Churchill Livingstone Elsevier; 208-222.

[20] Gott M, Galena E, Hinchliff S, Elford H (2004). Opening a can of worms: GP and practice nurse barriers to talking about sexual health in primary care. Family Practice 21: 528–536.

[21] Wendt E, Lidell E, Westersthael A, Marklund B, Hildingh C (2011). Young women's perceptions of being asked questions about sexuality and sexual abuse – a content analysis. Midwifery 27(2): 250-6.

[22] Pelvin B (2006). Life skills for midwifery practice. In: Pairman S, Pincombe J, Thorogood C, Tracy S, eds (2006). Midwifery: preparation for practice. Sydney: Churchill Livingstone Elsevier; 223-234.

[23] Riddick-Thomas NM (2009). Ethics in midwifery. In: Fraser DM, Cooper MA, eds. Myles textbook for midwives. 15th ed. Edinburgh: Churchill Livingstone, Elsevier; 55-66.

[24] Oxford dictionary (2014). Definition of sexology. Available at: http://www.oxforddictionaries.com/definition/english/sexology (23.7.2014).

[25] Kinsey Institute (2014). The definition of sexology. Available at: http://www.kinseyinstitute.org/resources/abtsexology.html (3.7.2014).

[26] Haeberle EJ (1995). Sexological training for health professionals. Nordisk Sexologi 3:193-211.

[27] WHO (1998). Gender and Health: Technical Paper. Women's Health and Development, Family and Reproductive Health.

[28] Hudson P, Omokanye S (2009). Contraception and sexual health. In: Fraser DM, Cooper MA, eds. Myles textbook for midwives. 15th ed. Edinburgh: Churchill Livingstone, Elsevier; 705-725.

[29] Stensson K, Sidenvall B, Heimer G (2005). Midwives' experiences of routine antenatal questioning relating to men's violence against women. Midwifery 21: 311–321.

[30] Haboubi NH, Lincoln N (2003). Views of health professionals on discussing sexual issues with patients. Disability and Rehabilitation 25: 291–296.

[31] Wendt E, Hildingh C, Lidell, E, Westerstaehl A, Baigi A, Marklund B (2007). Young women's sexual health and their views on dialogue with health professionals. Acta Obstetricia et Gynecologica Scandinavica 86: 590–595.

[32] Davies R (2006). Completing the midwife-woman partnership. In: Pairman S, Pincombe J, Thorogood C, Tracy S, eds. Midwifery: preparation for practice. Sydney: Churchill Livingstone Elsevier, 543-561.

[33] Weerakoon P, Jones MK, Pynor R, Kilburn-Watt E (2004). Allied health professional students' perceived level of comfort in clinical situations that have sexual connotations. Journal of Allied Health 33: 189–193.

[34] Skoberne M, Mivšek AP (2003). Izobraževanje babic v Evropski uniji: evropske in svetovne težnje za kakovost v babištvu. Obzornik zdravstvene nege 37(1): 13-21.

[35] Skoberne M (2003). Spremembe na področju babištva-babiške nege ob vstopu v EU. V: Funkcionalno izobraževanje – zbornik predavanj. Ljubljana: Zveza društev medicinskih sester in zdravstvenih tehnikov Slovenije, Sekcija medicinskih sester babic, 14-17.

[36] Stanek Zidarič T, Mivšek AP, Skoberne M, Skubic M, Zakšek T (2009). Babištvo: visokošolski strokovni študijski program prve stopnje. 1. izd. Ljubljana: Zdravstvena fakulteta.

[37] 1KA. Tool for web surveys. Available at: http://english.1ka.si/c/695/Kaj_je_1KA/?preid=632 (20.7.2014)

[38] Laerd dissertations (2014). Total population sampling. Available at: http://dissertation.laerd.com/total-population-sampling.php (25.7.2014)

[39] Moreira ED, Brock G, Glasser DB, Nicolosi A, Laumann EO, Paik A, Wang T, Gingell C; GSSAB Investigators' Group (2005). Help seeking behaviour for sexual problems: the global study of sexual attitudes and behaviours. International Journal of Clinical Practice 59: 6–16.

[40] Warenius LU, Faxelid EA, Chishimba PN, Musandu JO, Ong'any AA, Nissen EB (2006). Nurse-midwives' attitudes towards adolescent sexual and reproductive health needs in Kenya and Zambia. Reproductive Health Matters 14 (27): 119-28.

[41] Cronin A (2005). Gender and sexuality. In: Stewart M, ed. Pregnancy, birth and maternity care: feminist perspectives. Oxford: Book for midwives, 11-25.

[42] Milivojević Z (2008). Emocije: razumevanje čustev v psihoterapiji. Novi Sad: Psihopolis institut.

[43] Walker S, Davis G (2013). Learning at work and university: Midwifery students and sexual health advice. Practitioner Research in Higher Education Journal 7(1): 63-77.

[44] Amador JA, Miles L, Peters CB (2006). The practice of problem-based learning: a guide to implementing PBL in the college classroom. San Francisco : Anker.

[45] Guilbert JJ (2004). Didaktični priročnik za učitelje na zdravstvenih šolah. Maribor: Unigrafika.

[46] Marentič Požarnik B, Peklaj C (2002). Preverjanje in ocenjevanje za uspešnejši študij. Ljubljana: Center za pedagoško izobraževanje Filozofske fakultete.

[47] Lozar Manfreda K, Hlebec V, Vehovar V (2002). Web as questionnaire designing tool: Is there a limit? Available at: http://www.websm.org/index.php?fl=2&lact=8&vir=42 (1.8.2014)

[48] Vehovar V, Lozar Manfreda K (2008) Overview: online surveys. In: Fielding NG, Lee RM, Blank G, eds. The SAGE Handbook of Online Research Methods. London: Sage Publications, 177-94.

[49] Lozar Manfreda K, Bosnjak M, Berzelak J, Haas I, Vehovar V (2008). Web surveys versus other survey modes: a meta-analysis comparing response rates. Journal of the Market Research Society 50(1): 79.

Chapter 2

Raising Children for a Healthy Sexual Relationship in Adulthood

Anita Jug Došler

Additional information is available at the end of the chapter

http://dx.doi.org/10.5772/59084

1. Introduction

Parents want their children to grow up to be healthy, happy and financially secure adults. Part of this challenge includes raising a sexually healthy child, a responsibility that often isn't openly discussed and for which parents receive little, if any, expert guidance. Sexually healthy adults begin as children who are raised in sexually healthy families. In such a family, parents understand that teaching their children about sexuality is just as important as teaching them about safety, human values and healthy decision-making. Each member of a sexually healthy family is treated with dignity and respect, and family members can discuss sexual issues in a comfortable and frank manner [1]. When many people hear the word "sexuality", they often hear only the first syllable. Sexuality is not the same as sex. Sexuality includes everything that defines us as girls and boys, men and women. Teaching children about sexuality requires more than simply explaining anatomy and reproduction - it means talking to them about relationships, families, parenthood and good decision-making. Sexuality encompasses our physical development, sexual knowledge, attitudes, values and behaviours - it is shaped not solely by our biology and psychology, but also by our culture, family history, education and experiences [2].

On the basis of these recommendations, the following chapter presents the argument that raising children for a healthy sexual relationship in adulthood is one of the most important responsibilities of parents and one which has to start when our child is a newborn.

1.1. Background

As a parent, our responsibility for raising a sexually healthy child starts when our child is a newborn. How we touch, talk and play with our infant teaches him or her about gender roles and how to express emotion and affection [3]. Talking about sex and sexuality is key to raising sexually healthy children. It gives us an opportunity to send the right message and share our values and beliefs. Many characteristics of sexually healthy families are not explicitly about sex or sexuality, but are about how each member of the family interacts with each other. Sexually healthy parents demonstrate that they value, respect, accept and trust their children – and that they expect to be treated that way in return. They listen to their children and seriously try to understand their points of view. They regularly share their values, stay actively involved in their children's lives, and aren't afraid to set age-appropriate limits for behaviour [1]. It is important that parents let their children know that they can depend on them for honest, reliable answers. It is not always easy for parents to talk with their children about sexuality. We have to find out what our child already knows and after that correct the child regarding misinformation and give the true facts. As parents we have to use the conversation as an opportunity to convey our values[1] [2].

1.2. Sexual development and behaviour in young children

Like all forms of human development, sexual development begins at birth. Sexual development includes not only the physical changes that occur as children grow, but also the sexual knowledge and beliefs they come to learn and the behaviours they show. Any given child's sexual knowledge and behaviour is strongly influenced by the child's age, what the child observes (including the sexual behaviours of family and friends), and what the child is taught (including cultural and religious beliefs concerning sexuality and physical boundaries) [6]. As parents we have to know that sexuality includes many components which are equally important. They are: anatomy and reproductive health (biological sex, pregnancy, childbirth, hygiene, general health care, etc.); gender identity and gender roles (how we see ourselves as male or female, and what we are taught about the way men and women should act); relationships (behaviours, expectations, satisfaction, abuse, etc.); love and affection (how we express love and affection to friends, family, etc.); body image (how we feel about our bodies and needs); sexual orientation (physical and emotional attraction to a man, woman, or both); sensuality and pleasure (accepting and enjoying our own bodies and accepting and enjoying the bodies of our sexual partner(s); sexual activity (acts of intimacy such as hugging, kissing, touching, and sexual intercourse); sexual exploration and play (they are a natural part of childhood sexual development, and help children not only learn about their own bodies, but about the social and cultural rules that govern sexual behaviour) [4,5,6].

Very young and preschool-aged children (four or younger) are naturally immodest, and may display open and occasionally startling-curiosity about other people's bodies and bodily functions, such as touching women's breasts, or wanting to watch when grownups go to the bathroom. Wanting to be naked (even if others are not) and showing or touching private parts while in public are also common in young children. They are curious about their own bodies and may quickly discover that touching certain body parts feels nice (for more on what children typically do at this and other ages, see Table 1).

---

1 Our values are personal beliefs that affect how we think, feel and act. Values can change over time with new knowledge and life experiences. Some values that we want to teach our children may come easily to us because we feel strongly about them while others may need more thought [4].

http://dx.doi.org/10.5772/59084

Preschool children (less than four years)	• Exploring and touching private parts, in public and in private. • Rubbing private parts (with hand or against objects). • Showing private parts to others. • Trying to touch mother's or other women's breasts. • Removing clothes and wanting to be naked. • Attempting to see other people when they are naked or undressing (such as in the bathroom). • Asking questions about their own - and others'- bodies and bodily functions. • Talking to children their own age about bodily functions such as "poo" and "pee".
Young children (approximately four-six years)	• Purposefully touching private parts (masturbation), occasionally in the presence of others. • Attempting to see other people when they are naked or undressing. • Mimicking dating behaviour (such as kissing, or holding hands). • Talking about private parts and using "naughty" words, even when they don't understand the meaning. • Exploring private parts with children their own age (such as "playing doctor", "I'll show you mine if you show me yours," etc.).
School-aged children (approximately seven-12 years)	• Purposefully touching private parts (masturbation), usually in private. • Playing games with children their own age that involve sexual behaviour (such as "truth or dare", "playing family," or "boyfriend/girlfriend"). • Attempting to see other people naked or undressing. • Looking at pictures of naked or partially naked people. • Viewing/listening to sexual content in media (television, films, games, the Internet, music, etc.). • Wanting more privacy (for example, not wanting to undress in front of other people) and being reluctant to talk to adults about sexual issues. • Beginnings of sexual attraction to/interest in peers.

Table 1. Common sexual behaviours in childhood [6].

As children grow older and interact more with other children (approximately ages four–six), they become more aware of the differences between boys and girls, and more social in their exploration. In addition to exploring their own bodies through touching or rubbing their private parts (masturbation), they may begin "playing doctor" and copying adult behaviours such as kissing and holding hands. As children become increasingly aware of the social rules governing sexual behaviour and language (such as the importance of modesty or which words are considered "naughty"), they may try to test these rules by using naughty words. They may also ask more questions about sexual matters, such as where babies come from, and why boys and girls are physically different. Once children enter grade school (approximately ages seven–12), their awareness of social rules increases and they become more modest and want more privacy, particularly around adults. Although touching oneself (masturbation) and sexual play continue, children at this age are likely to hide these activities from adults. Curiosity about adult sexual behaviour increases particularly as puberty approaches and children may begin to seek out sexual content on television, in films, and in printed material. Telling jokes and "dirty" stories is common. Children approaching puberty are likely to start displaying romantic and sexual interest in their peers [6].

2. Milestones in the development of sexual conscience in children

Knowledge of what is typical at different ages helps adults understand the meaning of children's decisions in situations which present moral dilemmas. Parents who are warm and communicative with their children, starting at an early age, while still maintaining control in the form of limits, raise children who are more self-respecting, who are more socially competent, and who deal more effectively with problems. Children gradually develop the cognitive and emotional capacities that form the basis of knowing and feeling what is right and what is wrong and then acting in accordance with that knowledge. They need caring adults to help them. Feeling for the emotions of others is key to developing a sense of right and wrong; it emerges at an early age and needs to be nurtured in a caring environment [16].

The ways in which parents relate to their children falls into certain patterns, and finding the right balance is the key to helping children attain an internal sense of conscience and values for a healthy sexual relationship in adulthood. Research has identified basic parenting styles:

- When parents balance affection, warmth and respect with a firm level of control in the form of limit-setting, children are more likely to be self-respectful, to deal with problems, and to establish a sense of values, e.g., "We listen to your ideas and opinions as we develop family rules.". This parenting style is known as authoritative.
- When parents are overly indulgent children often struggle to learn the limits of what is acceptable and to develop their inner controls, e.g., "We will let you find yourself." This parenting style is known as permissive.
- When parents are too controlling and autocratic, e.g., "Do as I say because I say so.", children have difficulty in establishing their own control, sense of social responsibility and their own sense of moral values. This parenting style is known as authoritarian.

Below are some parenting suggestions that may prove helpful in finding the authoritative parent [14,16]:

- Be aware of your own needs and the ways in which your role as a parent is coloured by your relationship with your own parents.
- Monitor your own behaviour in the ordinary situations of daily life; children tune in when adults tell white lies, such as saying you are not at home to avoid certain people, writing an excusal note for school saying the child was sick, when s/he is really going to visit a relative.
- Model helpful and kind behaviours, such as assisting people in need, lending a hand, or giving up your seat to an older and/or handicapped person.

- Praise your child for unselfish acts.
- Point out the consequences of one's acts for others.
- Participate in positive activities such as community service, sports, music, all of which imbue children with a sense of purpose.
- Allow children to participate in decisions which affect the family.
- When discussing a child's behaviour, focus attention on the way in which the feelings of the other person are affected.

Parents model sexually healthy attitudes in their own relationships, and they are appropriately affectionate in front of their children [3]. We can help children grow to be sexually healthy adults by [1,4,6-10]:

- Using the correct words for body parts and functions to help children respect and take care of their bodies. You cannot predict when and what your child will ask, so don't worry if you don't know the answer - look up answers together.
- Using positive touch to give your children feelings of closeness, comfort, security and safety. For example, hold hands and give lots of cuddles and hugs.
- Sharing your values with your children. Knowing your values and explaining why they are important to you will help your children develop their own.
- Talking to your children about their responsibilities and the behaviours you expect.
- Teaching your children to think about what they say and do, and how their comments and actions make others feel.
- Use assertive communication to express feelings, resist pressure and protect themselves.
- Talking to your children about sexual abuse: what it is and how they can protect themselves.
- Giving your children equal opportunities and respect. Treating girls and boys differently can affect how capable they feel.
- Being a role model for what you want your child to learn.
- Introducing the topic. Don't wait for your child to start the conversation. Many parents put off talking to their children about sexuality, assuming that a child will ask when he wants to know something. Some children however are reluctant to begin these discussions, and others simply aren't the type who ask lots of questions. It is a parent's responsibility to introduce the topic, little by little. Your child might never ask, but s/he still needs to know.
- Listening to your child, be honest and talk about both your own and your child's feelings.
- Looking for teaching opportunities. Teaching opportunities arise naturally and provide a good avenue by which to talk about some aspects of sexuality or other important topics.
- Encouraging the child's critical thinking and reflection about gender identities and gender-role stereotyping. Since the media plays a major role in the sexual education of individuals,

effective sexual health education provides training in critical media literacy to help individuals identify and deconstruct hidden and overt sexual messages and stereotypes. Importantly, comprehensive sexual health education helps individuals to understand how these messages may affect their sexual health.

- It is never too early to help your children feel good about their individuality, their body image and their sexuality. Conveying these messages from the beginning will set them on the right track. Help them tell the difference between fact and fiction. Help them understand what is happening to their bodies.
- Talk to them about their feelings and their relationships. Share with children your opinions and what you believe in.

As we can see in Table 2 it is important to focus on the facts, your values and your child's responsibilities and self-esteem when handling sexual situations and questions. This four-point plan - a caring parent's guide - can help us respond to the questions your child might have about sexuality.

Acknowledge the facts.	• Answer honestly. Do your best to give accurate information and clarify any misconceptions. • Research the facts with your child if you don't know the answer.
Communicate your family values.	• Share what you believe in and what is important to you. • Be a good role model and show by example.
Emphasize your children's responsibilities.	• Make sure your expectations are clear. • Help them understand the possible negative consequences of their decisions and actions. • Help them develop assertive communication skills for resisting pressure and committing to their decisions when friends disagree.
Respect and promote your children's self-esteem.	• Be encouraging: help your children and teens feel good about themselves, their changing bodies and emotions. • Let them explore and share their thoughts and feelings about sexuality. • Treat them with respect and keep the lines of communication open.

Table 2. The four-point plan – a caring parent's guide [11].

The majority of families have both parents working outside the home; children are increasingly involved in extracurricular activities and spend more time out of adult supervision than ever before. Because of this, child-rearing experts state that we must do more to teach our children early in their lives about how to make good decisions and how to take appropriate actions. This teaching must cover all issues relevant to their lives, including difficult subjects such as sexuality and ways to relate positively to peers [12]. Approaches and methods effectively integrate the four key elements of sexual health education: (1) knowledge acquisition and understanding, (2) motivation and personal insight, (3) skills that support sexual health and (4) environments conducive to sexual health. Various sources of formal and informal sexual health education are created for diverse learning styles and are age-appropriate [8,12]. Parents have an obligation to create an open environment in which to start the conversation. Here are six steps to encourage your children to talk about difficult issues [4,6,12]:

First step

Foster an open environment: be available to listen to your children. This means letting them ask you anything or sound out any idea. Give them plenty of opportunities to start a discussion - tell them that you are always there for their questions or concerns. Don't criticize them for having questions, even if they raise ideas that are disturbing to you. Keep the lines of communication with your children open through small talk - often big ideas begin as little thoughts which are slipped into the middle of a conversation about something else. Finally, ask questions. One tip: use current events or situations on a favourite TV programme as an opener for a chat with your children and ask them for their opinions. Then listen attentively to your child's answer.

Second step

Give your undivided attention: when the opportunity for dialogue presents itself, focus your attention on the conversation and your child. Don't let other things distract you or divide your concentration. Turn off the television, let the answering machine pick up the ringing phone and sit down one-on-one with your child. If it is really a bad time to talk, schedule it for another time, but first make sure that waiting is okay with your child; and be sure to keep that appointment - there is nothing more disappointing to child than a forgotten meeting to discuss something of importance to them.

Third step

For important topics, start the talk: if you think it is difficult for an adult to raise certain topics, imagine how hard it must be for a child. Believe it or not, our children want us to talk with them, so look for moments during the day that seem ripe for conversation. Our conversations with our children should include:

- the importance of feeling good about oneself,
- the importance about how to have healthy, respectful relationships,
- the importance of clear messages from you about your values and expectations about sexual and other important personal decisions.

With this information, our children are better prepared to resist peer pressure and other influences and to make healthy decisions.

Fourth step

Talk with your kids on their level: children don't always get it when you speak to them in abstractions. Assess your own values before you talk to your children and think about the things that you value in your relationships. Give your children clear examples of what are appropriate manners. Talk to them about the standards of conduct that you expect in the way they talk and present themselves to others.

Fifth step

Speaking often and honestly with your child helps establish clear channels of communication early in your child's life. No one likes to be lectured, so try having many brief, yet insightful, conversations instead. Plus, frequent chats are a great way of communicating, reinforcing your values and letting your children know that you are interested in their lives. The outcome of growing and learning through open communication is the development of strong, emotionally complete men and women who are interested in and capable of having healthy relationships. Understand the questions and answer honestly: if you are not sure what your child is asking, say so. Once you understand the question, give an answer that you know is correct and honest. If you don't know the answer, say so and assure your child that you can research it and come up with a solution together. Teach your child problem solving and explain the »danger zone« to them.

Sixth step

All too often, children get the majority of their sexual education from other children and from media sources such as television shows, songs, movies, and video games. Not only is this information often wrong, it may have very little to do with the sexual values that parents want to convey. Explicit adult sexual activities are sometimes found during "family time" television shows, in commercials, and on cartoon/children's channels, and can have an influence on children's behaviours. Controlling media exposure and providing appropriate alternatives is an important part of teaching children about sexual issues. Get to know the rating systems of games, movies and television shows, and make use of the parental controls available through many Internet, cable, and satellite providers. However, don't assume that just by activating those controls you will be taking care of the situation. It is very important for you to be aware of what your children are watching on television and online, and make time to watch television with them. When appropriate, you can use this time as a springboard to talk about sexual or relationship issues, and to help children develop the skills to make healthy decisions about their behaviour and relationships.

As your child becomes older, you will continue to teach him or her about sexuality, through role-modelling and verbal communication as well as body language. For example, if your child starts playing with his or her genitals while sitting on the toilet, how you respond sends a message that may affect his or her body image in a positive or negative manner. If you get upset or show anger, your child may get the idea that the genitals are a bad or dirty part of the body [13-14].

By remaining calm and not avoiding the question, you are sending your child the message that you are open to talking about sexuality. A lot of parents worry more about exactly what they will say when asked a sexuality question, instead of how to say it. When answering your child's question, be sure to give your child accurate information while also letting him or her know your views and values. Keep your answers brief and uncomplicated. Start with a simple answer and give your child more information if he or she continues to ask more questions. Normalize and validate the child's question and then ask the child why he or she is asking you this question. This step reassures the child that his or her question is normal. It will also give you a sense of what caused your child to ask that question and from where he or she is getting information. You can also ask your child what he or she thinks the answer is. It is important to provide information that is appropriate to the child's age and developmental level.

In Table 3, you will find an overview of some of the most important information and safety messages for children at various ages. Keep in mind that you do not need to bombard children with information all at once. Let the situation - and the child's questions - guide the lessons you share. The important thing is to let children know that you are ready to listen and to answer whatever questions they may have [13-14].

Preschool children (less than four years)	• Basic information. • Boys and girls are different. • Accurate names for body parts of boys and girls. • Babies come from mummies. • Rules about personal boundaries (for example, keeping private parts covered, not touching other children's private parts). • Give simple answers to all questions about the body and bodily functions. • The difference between "okay" touches (which are comforting, pleasant, and welcome) and "not okay" touches (which are intrusive, uncomfortable, unwanted, or painful). • Your body belongs to you. • Everyone has the right to say "no" to being touched, even by grownups. • No child or adult has the right to touch your private parts. • It is okay to say "no" when grownups ask you to do things that are wrong, such as touching private parts or keeping secrets from Mummy or Daddy. • There is a difference between a "surprise" - which is something that will be revealed sometime soon, like a present - and a "secret," which is something you are never supposed to tell. • Stress that it is never okay to keep secrets from Mummy and Daddy. • Who to tell if people do "not okay" things to you, or ask you to do "not okay" things to them.
Young children (approximately four-six years)	• Boys' and girls' bodies change when they get older. • Simple explanations of how babies grow in their mothers' wombs and about the birth process.

	• Rules about personal boundaries (such as, keeping private parts covered, not touching other children's private parts). • Simple answers to all questions about the body and bodily functions. • Touching your own private parts can feel nice, but is something done in private. • Sexual abuse is when someone touches your private parts or asks you to touch their private parts. • It is sexual abuse even if it is by someone you know. • Sexual abuse is never the child's fault. • If a stranger tries to get you to go with him or her, run and tell a parent, teacher, neighbour, police officer, or other trusted adult. • Who to tell if people do "not okay" things to you, or ask you to do "not okay" things to them.
School-aged children (approximately seven-12 years)	• What to expect and how to cope with the changes of puberty (including menstruation and wet dreams). • Basics of reproduction, pregnancy, and childbirth. • Risks of sexual activity (pregnancy, sexually transmitted diseases). • Basics of contraception. • Masturbation is common and not associated with long-term problems but should be done in private. • Sexual abuse may or may not involve touch. • How to maintain safety and personal boundaries when chatting or meeting people online. • How to recognize and avoid risky social situations. • Dating rules.

Table 3. What to teach when [1,4,9-10,15].

3. Conclusion

Preparing children for puberty before they begin to develop makes it easier for them to make the transition. It also helps you to get in touch with the fact that one day your "baby" will start to look more like an adult. Through the article we have shown that children are more likely to abstain if they have high self-esteem and goals for the future. Acknowledge the ways in which your children are special and wonderful, help them to develop their talents and skills, emphasize the importance of education, encourage them to take healthy risks like trying out for a sports team or running for student government, and work with them on a plan to achieve their goals [4,14]. After considering all that makes up sexuality, it is easy to see how talking

http://dx.doi.org/10.5772/59084

and teaching about sexuality should not be limited to a one-time event. Talking and teaching about sexuality is a lifelong and ongoing process. Throughout this process, each person develops attitudes and values that guide choices, relationships and understanding.

Author details

Anita Jug Došler

Address all correspondence to: anita.jug@zf.uni-lj.si

Faculty of Health Sciences, Ljubljana, Midwifery Department, Slovenia

References

[1] Haffner DW. From diapers to dating: A parent's guide to raising sexually healthy children - from infancy to middle school. New York: Newmarket Press; 2008.

[2] Changes in me: A resource for educators on puberty and adolescent development. Healthy sexuality program. Peel Public Health; 2011. https://www.peelregion.ca/health/commhlth/bodyimg/changes-in-me/pdf/ChangesInMe.pdf (accessed 26 May 2014).

[3] MacPherson KC. Is childhood becoming oversexed? Post-Gazette National Bureau 2005:1-2. http://old.post-gazette.com/pg/05128/500945.stm (accessed 26 May 2014).

[4] Adamson D, Clemente A, Little W, Moody L, Simms M, Bayley M. Hej, What do I say. A parent to parent guide on how to talk to children about sexuality. New York: Margaret Sanger Square; 2009.

[5] Understanding and Coping with Sexual Behavior Problems in Children. The National Child Traumatic Stress Network: Child Sexual Abuse Committee and National Center on Sexual Behavior of Youth; 2009. http://nctsn.org/nctsn_assets/pdfs/caring/sexualdevelopmentandbehavior.pdf (accessed 16 June 2014).

[6] Raising Healthy Kids: Families Talk about Sexual Health. Advocates for youth. http://www.advocatesforyouth.org/parents/180?task=view (accessed 26 may 2014).

[7] Healthy sexuality. Peel Public Health. http://www.peelregion.ca/health/sexuality/relations/comm-assert.htm (accessed 26 May 2014).

[8] Canadian Guidelines for Sexual Health Education. Canada: Public Health Agency of Canada; 2008.

[9] Haffner DW. From Diapers to Dating: A Parent's Guide to Raising Sexually Healthy Children From Infancy to Middle School. New York: Newmarket Press; 2000.

[10] Hickling M. The New Speaking Of Sex: What Your Children Need To Know And When They Need To Know It. New York: Northstone Publishing; 2005.

[11] Lipton M, Weber SJ. Sexuality Education at Home: The Caring Parent's Guide, The Pacific Coast Centre of Sexology. Vancouver: British Columbia; 1999.

[12] Claiborne L. Parent's handbook: How to talk to your children about developing healthy relationships. New York: The Parenting Institute, NYU Child Study; 1998. http://www.aboutourkids.org/files/pages/assets/Liz_Claiborne_Handbook.pdf (accessed 26 May 2014).

[13] Logan Levkoff MS. Third Base Ain't What It Used to Be: What Your Kids Are Learning about Sex Today—and How to Teach Them to Be Sexually Healthy Adults. New York: New American Library; 2007.

[14] Richardson J, Schuster M. Everything You Never Wanted Your Kids to Know about Sex (But Were Afraid They'd Ask): The Secrets to Surviving Your Child's Sexual Development from Birth to the Teens. New York: Three Rivers Press; 2004.

[15] Hagan JF, Shaw JS, Duncan P. Promoting healthy sexual development and sexuality. In bright futures: Guidelines for health supervision of infants, children and adolescents. Elk Grove Village, IL: American Academy of Pediatrics; 2008. http://www.ewidgetsonline.net/dxreader/Reader.aspx?token=d316YO0Z3HhU±Gof2cp8IA%3d%3d&rand=671109678&buyNowLink=&page=&chapter= (accessed 16 June 2014).

[16] Gurian A. Learning Right from Wrong. CSC Letter 2005; 10(2) 1-4.

Chapter 3

Promotion and Health Education for Healthy Sexuality

Andreja Kvas

Additional information is available at the end of the chapter

http://dx.doi.org/10.5772/60140

1. Introduction

Health promotion is a broad concept that can be interpreted differently by different disciplines since numerous health-oriented activities, which are based on different philosophies, can be found under this term [1]. The history and development of the health promotion movement can be traced back to seven conferences for health promotion held in Ottawa (1986), Adelaide (1988), Sundsvall (1991), Jakarta (1997), Mexico (2000), Bangkok (2005) and Helsinki (2013) [2]. The most important historical milestone for health promotion was the first international conference in Ottawa, where the Ottawa Charter introduced the concept of citizen empowerment, the need for multi-sectoral and multi-agency operations, the media as one of the key promoters of health and the decentralization of health promotion in a manner that involves more active involvement of people in the implementation of strategies for health promotion at the local and community levels [3]. Within the context of health promotion, we are attempting to have an impact on individuals and the community so that they care for, maintain and strengthen their health. Health should be seen in conjunction with the natural and social environments in which people live and work, so the "Ottawa Charter for Health Promotion" defined the creation of environments that depict health as a priority area and an important value and is striving to create conditions for healthy choices (supportive environments) [4].

Health promotion in practice utilizes seven key strategic approaches: health communication, health education, self-help and mutual assistance, community development and mobilization, advocacy and policy development [1]. Health education is a component of health promotion and not a synonym for it. Health professionals often equated the concept of health education with health promotion [5, 6, 7]. Health promotion is a versatile social and political process, involving not only activities aimed at strengthening the skills and abilities of people but also activities aimed at changing social, environmental and economic circumstances so as to mitigate their impact on the health of both individuals and communities [1]. The purpose of health education is to help people assume a healthy lifestyle, motivate them to this end and enable them to become actively involved in the care of their health [8]. Through health education, we improve both individual and community knowledge as well as values and skills to ensure effective action in the direction of health [9].

In the context of health promotion and health education, midwives act as promoters of healthy sexuality, being the ones that help people adopt and maintain healthy sexual behaviour. Healthy sexuality is a topic to which sufficient time must be devoted already in early childhood which should continue and be supplemented all the way up to late old age. Sexuality is an important part of a person's life throughout the entire life cycle and, thus, may promote or inhibit the development of personal identity, well-being and health [10, 11]. People experience sex very subjectively because it is associated with love and anger, with tenderness and aggression, with intimacy and adventure, and with pleasure and pain [12]. In society, the subject of sex has always been taboo which is spoken of "quietly" [13]. It is a topic that is strongly linked to the individual's intimacy; therefore, the manner in which the midwife explains healthy sexuality is very important. Numerous definitions exist regarding what healthy sexuality is. "The definition of sexuality includes many components including (but not limited to): sexual attitudes, sexual desires, sexual behaviours engaged in, sexual preferences, sexual identification, and sexual function" [14]. The World Health Organization (WHO) defines healthy sexuality as "a state of physical, emotional, mental and social well-being in relation to sexuality; it is not merely the absence of disease, dysfunction or infirmity. Sexual health requires a positive and respectful approach to sexuality and sexual relationships, as well as the possibility of having pleasurable and safe sexual experiences, free of coercion, discrimination and violence. For sexual health to be attained and maintained, the sexual rights of all persons must be respected, protected and fulfilled" [15].

If the midwife finds that a person's life does not include healthy sexuality, she can assist the individual in changing risky sexual behaviour. Theories and models of individual health behaviour can prove helpful, such as the health belief model (HBM), theory of reasoned action (TRA), theory of planned behaviour (TPB), integrated behavioural model, transtheoretical model and stages of change (TTM), and precaution adoption process model.

This chapter will present the health education for the individual or couple in a more comprehensive manner using the transtheoretical model and stages of change and prior determination of his/her health literacy.

2. Methodology

A literature review was performed. Literature found with the aid of the information service EBSCOhost using the databases CINAHL (Cumulative Index to Nursing and Allied Health Literature) and MEDLINE was used. The following keywords using Boolean operators (AND, OR) in various combinations were used: healthy sexuality, health education, health promotion communication, midwifery, motivational interviewing, motivation, patient, health behaviour change, theory change, a model of change. To narrow down the search for literature, we chose: the English language, scientific journals, available extracts, available full-length articles and the past ten-year period (2004– 2014). We also utilized earlier literature for explaining the terms, definitions and results of some studies. The search for literature was conducted from June 2014 to November 2014.

3. Literature review

Gynaecological examination is a common intervention in reproductive health care and may present an opportunity for midwives with the help of a conversation (dialogue) to promote the healthy sexuality of women [11, 16]. The midwife can carry out a conversation either before or after a gynaecological examination/intervention. The midwife should reserve time for a conversation, be well prepared for it and conduct it in a location where nothing will disturb them (without people entering the room). Over the course of the conversation, the midwife will be able to determine the sexual behaviour of the individual – whether that individual has any problems they would like to discuss. If the midwife determines deviations in the sexual behaviour of the individual [17], she should, together with the individual, create a plan to change the individual's behaviour using the transtheoretical model of behaviour change. It is important to establish a good dialogue that gives the individual an opportunity to tell and receive answers from the midwife and allows them to reflect on their sexual health and life situations [18]. In doing so, the midwife should let the individual know that they can confide in her without feeling guilty, afraid or ashamed [19].

The basis for effective and quality implementation of health education is to determine the health literacy of the individual. This can be determined on the basis of a conversation with the individual and with the aid of various questionnaires to assess health and specific literacy, for example the Test of Functional Health Literacy in Adults (TOFHLA) [20], the Rapid Estimate of Adult Literacy in Medicine (REALM) [21], the Nutritional Literacy Scale (NLS) [22] and the Literacy Assessment for Diabetes (LAD) scale [23].

3.1. Health literacy

Health literacy, a priority in health promotion initiatives, is a pillar of modern life and one of the bases of individual health. A growing belief is that healthcare professionals should take into account the level of health literacy of individuals in order to adapt interventions and to optimize their impact [24]. Health literacy is a stronger predictor of the health status of an individual than income, employment status, education level, or racial and ethnic group [15]. Individual health literacy may vary depending on the health problems of the individual, the healthcare provider and the system that provides health care [25, 26]. Health literacy is the ability to access, understand, evaluate and communicate information as a way of promoting, maintaining and improving health in a variety of environments based on life stages [27]. This definition of health literacy shows what influences the medical decisions of individuals regarding themselves and others in everyday life [28].

Health literacy need to address in a broader sense than simply becoming informed and reading pamphlets and brochures, and the proper selection of health services [29]. Health literacy comprises the skills and knowledge necessary for understanding diseases and treatment, as well as the capability for efficient orientation and functioning within the health system [30]. Health literacy is a cognitive and social skill which determines the individual's motivation and ability to obtain access to information and to understand them and use them to improve and maintain their health [29].

Health literacy for the individual includes the search for timely and proper medical care, proper taking of medication and understanding of given instructions. It is the capability of the individual to understand instructions and properly introduce the information received into everyday life [31].

In the health care system, health literacy refers to the following: 1) the expression of an individual's needs, signs and symptoms ; 2) the identification of health services and when to seek them; 3) the use of resources in a complex health care system; 4) how to act when cooperating with health professionals; 5) the ability to understand the recommendations of health professionals and the rights and responsibilities of the individual; and 6) the ability to adopt measures to improve their own health and safety, including that which is necessary for individual treatment and optimum use of equipment or medication [24, 32, 33].

Health literacy, a priority in health promotion initiatives, is a pillar of modern life and one of the bases of individual health. A growing belief is that healthcare professionals should take into account the level of health literacy of individuals in order to adapt interventions and to optimize their impact [24].

3.1.1. Studies on the impact of health literacy

Researchers have established limited health literacy to be quite common. Compared to general literacy, health literacy can be measured at the individual, organizational, community and population levels. Research by the European Health Literacy Survey showed that 12% of all respondents were generally inadequately health literate, while 35% possessed problems regarding health literacy, so this is not just a problem of minority populations [15].

The low level of health literacy is associated with more frequent visits to emergency medical care, as well as more frequent and prolonged hospitalization [26]. Low health literacy not only affects the individual's health and development but also has great economical, social and cultural consequences. The research also stated that personal limiting factors, such as advanced age (over 65 years), low education, another native language or culture (recent immigrant), unemployment, low income, lack of daily reading and learning disorders, also affect health literacy [24]. The high level of health literacy is associated with improved ability of self-sufficiency of the population, results in more adequate supervision and control of chronic diseases and increased accessibility to and appropriate use of health services at a lower cost of operation of the health care system, and is also due to decreased use of other services and results in improved health outcomes [34, 35, 36].

Low health literacy is a widespread problem in the USA and affects approximately 40% of adults [37]. Studies in the USA have shown low health literacy to be associated with low self-initiative [25, 38] and fewer visits to the doctor [38, 39]. The use of complex medical terminology can lead to poor communication between doctors and patients [38, 40]. Patients with low health literacy find it harder to understand medical prescriptions [40]; patients possess limited skills in self-managing disease [41], leading to a higher incidence of hospitalization [25, 38] and higher mortality [31, 42].

In the Czech Republic, based on a sample of pregnant women (n = 360), the key determinants that affect their health literacy were found. Health literacy and healthier lifestyle of pregnant women are associated with a higher level of education and long-term contact with a midwife in prenatal courses. These participants reported that they were better prepared overall for labour and birth and felt less stressed at the end of pregnancy, with a number of them opting for breastfeeding. Professional intervention and advice on primary prevention topics are necessary to achieve goals such as decreased smoking, alcohol consumption and bad nutritional habits, and improved support and skills for coping with stress. These enlightened and well-educated women clearly stated that the information provided to them by midwives helped them manage the postnatal period and that they plan to be in contact with midwives during future pregnancies [43].

In some countries in Africa, health literacy, especially among women, is especially low because they do not know how to read and write. Thus, the level of health literacy in South Africa and Zimbabwe is close to 80%, while in the poorest countries, such as Nigeria and Burkina Faso, only 10% of the women know how to read and write. Health literacy among women in these countries can be raised only through a greater involvement of young girls in education [44].

3.2. Health promotion and health education

Health promotion represents a comprehensive social and political process; it not only embraces actions directed at strengthening the skills and capabilities of individuals but also actions directed towards changing social, environmental and economic conditions so as to alleviate their impact on public and individual health. Health promotion is the process of enabling people to increase control over the determinants of their health and there by improve their health [45]. It focuses primarily on those determinants of the natural (air, water, soil, food and immediate living conditions) and social environments (social networking, social exclusion and health inequality) which one has the power to influence. At the forefront on the one hand are the health- risk behaviours of individuals, such as smoking, an unbalanced diet, lack of physical activity, alcohol abuse and illicit drugs, elevated blood lipid and blood sugar levels, obesity and stress [46, 47].

Health promotion enables individuals or groups to increase control over their own health by maintaining and improving it [48]. Health thus becomes a condition for everyday life, not just the result of life since the individual or community can identify and fulfil expectations, satisfy needs and to adapt to and manage the environment [49]. Some, due to such classifications, actually see the essence of health promotion in the empowerment of individuals to resist the industry which is selling them bad products; for example, they stop buying overly sweet or fatty foods that have adverse effects on their health. Nevertheless, individuals though well informed and even those for whom health represents a fundamental value do not always act in accordance [3].

Health promotion is not the exclusive responsibility of health professionals. Many agencies or entities are involved: education, employment, housing, transport and social services, as well as the individuals themselves [50]. It includes primary, secondary and tertiary prevention. Primary prevention consists of action that prevents disease or disability before it occurs. Secondary prevention comprises action related to early detection and treatment of disease. Tertiary prevention consists of action to avoid needless progression or complications of disease [50, 51].

Research shows that people find it very difficult to abandon unhealthy lifestyles (risky behaviours). Health professionals can achieve a great deal in this area within the scope of health education by implementing activities to change individual behaviour in schools, workplaces, hospitals and local communities. These activities include topics such as healthy diets, physical activity, prevention of smoking, mental health, prevention of infectious diseases, etc. [52]. Health education focuses on building the capacity of individuals through education, motivation, and the enhancement of skills and techniques to raise individual awareness for a healthy life. The health literacy of individuals is the result of effective health education which increases the capacity of individuals to access and use health information in adopting appropriate decisions on health and maintaining basic health [47, 52].

The major factors relating to health education are the voluntary cooperation of individuals and determination of their own health practices [53]. The individual should not have the feeling that health professionals want to push them into anything at any price. The process of learning and obtaining experience must be designed together with the individual using a variety of methods, such as individual learning, counselling, and encouragement to change their behaviour and habits [54, 55]. The aim of health education actions is primarily to change already- established behaviour and often to introduce new lifestyle habits and behaviours that will contribute to improving the health status of an individual [56]. Health education also plays a role in the prevention of disease, in health promotion, in the recognition and treatment of a disease, and in rehabilitation [57]. Health education is a constituent part of nursing and midwifery. It is important to take into account that we, healthcare professionals, are not the ones making the decisions in the process of health education and counselling and transmitting information to the individual. More effective are strategies where the individual decides what to do regarding behavioural changes [58].

Implementers of health education are also known as health educators. Health educators apply theories and models of health education in a targeted manner; they incorporate concepts of cooperation, encourage voluntary changes in the individual, incorporate health literacy and strengthen the capacity of individuals within health programmes and services, and they are important and indispensable members of the health promotion team [52]. It is important that health educators begin with health education early enough. Health education should already be introduced in the schooling period because children form their positions, values and attitudes at a very early age. People's habits and behaviours change considerably during the course of their lives. Even adults will often decide to change an unhealthy lifestyle [59], so health education is an important part of lifelong learning and accompanies people throughout their lives. Within the context of health education, children particularly acquire new patterns of healthy behaviour, while in adults, it most often regards the cessation of risky behaviours and habits that negatively affect the individual's health.

It is important that the midwife together with the individual plans the course of health education: when, where, how and in what way health education will take place [50]. The implementation of health education itself can be carried out based on the learning process, which is divided into four stages: assessment of learning needs (goals), preparation for achieving them (planning), implementation of teaching plans and evaluation of health teaching. Throughout all the stages of the health education process, it is important that the midwife monitors the mode of communication with individuals to enable her to obtain all necessary information concerning the individual's sexual behaviour. Based on the information obtained, the midwife, together with the individual, in the event of deviations in sexual behaviour will be able to develop a plan of health education to eliminate the risky behaviour.

3.2.1. The importance of communication in working with individuals

Communication is something we do all the time, whether we want to or not. We can avoid meeting others when we are not in the mood; nevertheless, we are still communicating. We cannot keep ourselves from communicating, even if we attempt not to talk to others [60]. Health professionals cannot perform their duties within the context of health promotion, such as providing physical and emotional support and information, without communicating with their patients [61, 62, 63]. Communication is a dynamic process and is influenced by social, cultural, ethical, economic, legal and technological factors [64].

Communication is the most important component of our work, for everything we do depends on communication [65, 66]. It is the foundation of our interaction with people. Communication enables a good and efficient exchange of information between people [65]. Good communication allows for the establishment of a genuine, relaxed relationship between health professionals and patients [66]. Everything we do with others comprises communication [67]. The ability to communicate is of vital importance for people, and through effective and open communication, the midwife can acquire the individual's trust and respect [68].

We are familiar with verbal and non-verbal communication [66, 69]. Verbal communication is used to transfer messages and also to establish relationships and empathy. Non-verbal communication includes behaviours that convey a message without the use of verbal language (touch, eye contact, gestures, posture, etc.) [66]. It is important that we establish a relationship of trust with individuals. Health professionals need to obtain the individual's trust and should in no way "buy" or demand it. In order to acquire a trusting relationship, health professionals must first establish a relationship based on respect with the other party. In addition, it is very important that health professionals transfer their expertise to patients in a manner that they will understand while not forgetting that they themselves are just people. When individuals ask us things, we should attempt to answer every question and, if necessary, turn to other professionals for advice. Each answer must be honest and never fake. In the process of communicating with patients, we should act in the way we want others to treat us [65].

When transferring a message, the words themselves hold little meaning, only 7%. A total of 55% of messages regard social significance and are the result of body language and facial expression, while the remainder 38% are derived from paralanguage, which includes tone, strength and colour of the voice [70]. Non-verbal communication comprises kinaesthetics (body movement), gestures, facial expressions, external appearance (clothing, jewellery and other accessories), paralanguage (communicative value of the voice) and time (duration of the event, intervals between events or sequence of events) [71]. For a proper understanding of non-verbal communication, one should consider the following: an error in reading body language is made if we interpret each gesture separately from each other or from the circumstances. Like spoken language, body language also comprises words, phrases and punctuation. For a proper understanding, body language needs to be seen as a series or group of gestures. Gestures should be studied in relation to the circumstances in which they occur [72].

The entire purpose of communication is to be express and exchange information, be comprehensible and to reach a mutual understanding [73]. One should be familiar with the four elements of open communication to ensure good communication: openness, timeliness, accuracy and comprehension. All these elements have a significant impact on the effectiveness of communication [74]. Effective communication is possible only if the recipient understands the information provided by the person transmitting it [17]. When communicating, we collaborate with others by listening, considering and hearing [67]. Listening can be defined as the art of capturing the true essence of the sender's message. In this case, the art means skill and ability [73]. When listening, one must observe the four main components of listening, as stages: the focus of attention, passive listening, paraphrasing and active listening [67]. It is important to mentally prepare ourselves so that we focus all our attention on our conversation partner. With passive listening, we further encourage our conversation partner to open up and express their concerns and ideas and describe the problem. Silence is very appropriate in doing so [67], because we do not always need to speak and silence always has priority over words [65]. More efficient than asking questions is encouraging the other person to clarify and provide more details while paraphrasing and actively listening. Particularly challenging is the skill of active listening, where we repeat the key points of the message by summarizing the statements of the other person, as is typical for paraphrasing, while also capturing what was not said. Active listening is mirroring contents and emotions [67, 73] and a reflection of feelings, including those that are concealed [73].

We should never judge interlocutors (patients) or caution them of the things that they have done. During the conversation, we should avoid medical terms, because all patients will not understand them and they may only confuse them. It is a good practice to put ourselves in the shoes of the patient so as to see the world through their eyes, making it easier to understand how the patient is experiencing and feeling the disease, treatment and rehabilitation. We should always ask the patient for their opinion. Never force the patient into the decision that seems most correct to us [65].

Communication between health professionals and patients should be assertive, and we define as firm, honest and respectful communication that which at the same time comprises responsible and mature behaviour where we assume full responsibility for our actions and behaviour [75]. Assertive communication is a self-expression for the defence of human personal rights, without violating the rights of others, and self-expression which allows for the different opinions and desires of others. In addition, health care professionals must ensure that they supply information which is supported by evidence through a number of sources such as various professional and scientific articles, books and videos and must support individuals by providing advice over telephone [76].

It is important that in their work, doctors, nurses, midwives, psychologists, social workers and physiotherapists master the skills of good communication and not only skills from their area of expertise [65]. As good communicators, they should respect the individuals. They should understand that in front of them is a person who has opinions, views and feelings; the individual may also be a person who comes from a different cultural environment, which should not adversely affect their communication [65, 77].

Good and effective communication is essential in the process of changing behaviours related to health. Models of individual health behaviour and models of interpersonal health behaviour can be used to change risky behaviours within the health education process. The transtheoretical model, a model involving individual health behaviour, will be presented in more detail later in the chapter.

3.3. Behavioural theories of change connected to health

To help in the development, management and evaluation of health education interventions, midwives and other health care professionals use a variety of design models based on health behavioural theories, such as the health belief model, theory of reasoned action, theory of planned behaviour, the transtheoretical model and stages of change, and the precaution adoption process model.

The health belief model (HBM) was developed in the 1950s by three social psychologists working in the public health field in the U SA (US Public Health Services) [1, 78]. The model focuses on the individual's attitude to health and their beliefs regarding health [57]. According to this model, the health behaviour of an individual depends on the degree of perceived health threats and judgements that a certain behaviour will be effective in reducing those threats [1, 78]. The application of HBM in practice has a positive impact on improving the health of the individual (e.g. regular condom use, regular physical activity). It is used at the individual level (one on one) and at the social level (legislation, changes in the physical environment) [57]. The theory of reasoned action (TRA) was developed by Icek Ajzen and Martin Fishbein. TRA says that health behaviours are the direct result of behavioural intentions (obligation to one's self and others), which are dependent on the actions and subjective norms regarding their adequacy. Subjective norms are derived from individual beliefs about what others think they should have done and the motivation to comply with them [1, 79, 80]. Later, Ajzen and his colleagues transformed the theory into the theory of planned behaviour (TPB), which in addition to the previously mentioned factors emphasizes that perceived behavioural control over a given action is required for the prediction of behaviour [1, 79]. TPB also includes motivational factors that indicate the extent a person is willing to take the new behaviour into account and how much effort they must invest to arrive at the desired result. TRA and TPB have been used to predict behaviour in a number of settings [81, 82]. The precaution adoption process model is a preventive behaviour model. It comprises the stages of cognitive processes that an individual must go through to be able to change their behaviour. The model seeks to identify all the stages involved when people commence health-protective behaviours and to determine the factors that lead people to move from one stage to the next [83, 84].

The transtheoretical model and stages of change (TTM) is described in the following text, the use of which allows health professionals to establish why people fail to change unhealthy lifestyles, helps them identify what information is necessary for people to develop effective strategies to deal with a change in behaviour and provides an insight into how to design prevention programmes that are successful [85, 86, 87]. TTM developed from a comparative analysis of the leading theories of psychotherapy and behaviour modification in an effort to agglomerate an area which is fragmented in more than 300 theories of psychotherapy [87, 88]. The impetus for the model arose when Prochaska and his colleagues conducted a comparative analysis among smokers who undertook change of their own initiative and those undertaking professional treatment. They identified ten processes of change that are predictive of successful smoking cessation in these sample populations. They estimated how often the groups used any of the ten processes [87, 89]. The participants used different processes during different time periods in their fight against smoking. The authors found that behaviour change takes place over several stages [85, 87, 90, 91]. The individuals pass through the stages during the change process, from precontemplation to maintaining the changes [87, 89, 92]. During each stage, the individual experiences different feelings and thoughts and establishes that various activities help to achieve the change. This change model is almost always presented in the form of a circle or a spiral [87, 93].

3.3.1. Core construct theories

The core construct theories of TTM are presented in Table 1.

Constructs	Description
Stages of change	
Precontemplation	No intention to take action with in the next 6 months.
Contemplation	Intends to take action within the next 6 months.
Preparation	Intends to take action within the next 30 days and has taken some behavioural steps in this direction.
Action	Changed overt behaviour for less than 6 months.
Maintenance	Changed overt behaviour for more than 6 months.
Termination	No temptation to relapse and 100 % confidence.
Processes of change	
Consciousness raising	Finding and learning new facts, ideas and tips that support the healthy behaviour change.
Dramatic relief	Experiencing the negative emotions (fear, anxiety, worry) that go along with unhealthy behavioural risks.

Constructs	Description
Self-reevaluation	Realizing that the behaviour change is an important part of one's identity as a person.
Environmental reevaluation	Realizing the negative impact of the unhealthy behaviour or the positive impact of the healthy behaviour one one's proximal social and/or physical environment.
Self-liberation	Making a firm commitment to change.
Helping relationship	Seeking and using support for the healthy behaviour change.
Counterconditioning	Substitution of healthier alternative behaviours and cognitions for the unhealthy behaviour.
Reinforcement management	Increasing the rewards for the positive behaviour change and decreasing the rewards for the unhealthy behaviour.
Stimulus control	Removing reminders or cues to engage in the unhealthy behaviour and adding cues or reminders to engage in the healthy behaviour.
Social liberation	Realizing that the social norms and changing in the direction of supporting the behaviour change.eh
Decisional balance	
Pros	Benefits of changing.
Cons	Costs of changing.
Self-efficacy	
Confidence	Confidence that one can engage in the healthy behaviour across different challenging situations.
Temptation	Temptation to engage in the unhealthy behaviour across different challenging situations.

Table 1. Transtheoretical Model Constructs [87].

3.3.2. *Stages of change*

In the past, a change in behaviour, such as quitting smoking, drinking or eating, was often constructed as an event. In TTM, researches identify three classes of variables: the stages of change, dependent variables (decisional balance and self-efficacy) and independent variables (the processes of change) [93, 94]. TTM represents change as a process that takes place over time, with progression through a sequence of six stages, although often not implemented in a straight line [87]. The individual goes through a series of stages with regard to their readiness to change: *precontemplation* where the individual does not intend to take action in the near future, *contemplation* where the individual has the intention of taking action in the next six months, *preparation* where the individual has the intention of taking action in the next 30 days, *action* where there is a permanent change in behaviour for six months or less and *maintenance* where the change lasts for more than six months. During the stages of change, individuals often return to a previous stage before achieving a lasting change in behaviour [89, 95]. People in the *termination* stage are no longer tempted and are confident that they will not return to the old unhealthy behaviour, even if they are depressed, anxious, bored, lonely, angry or stressed out [87].

Precontemplation, where there is no interest to change, is the stage when people do not intend to take action in the near future, which is usually measured in the subsequent six months. People can find themselves in this state because they are uninformed or under-informed about the consequences of their behaviour. Another reason is that they have tried many times to change the behaviour and have begun to doubt their ability to change. Both groups usually avoid reading, conversation or thoughts regarding their high-risk behaviour [87]. The person sees only the advantages of their current state and has no interest in changing their behaviour [88, 96]. These people are often labelled as rebellious or unmotivated or unprepared for health promotion programmes. The question is whether traditional health promotion programmes are ready for such individuals and whether they are motivated enough to adapt to the needs of the programmes [87].

In the *contemplation* stage, people intend to change their behaviour in the next six months [87, 93]. They are more aware of the benefits of change than those in the stage where they are not interested in change, but at the same time, they are also aware of the disadvantages arising from a change in behaviour [87]. This balance between the price of the change and its benefits can lead to a deep ambivalence with people remaining in the contemplation stage for a very long time, possibly for years, because they still have plenty of reasons to continue the current behaviour [88, 96]. Such persons are not prepared for traditionally oriented programmes which expect immediate action from individuals [87].

In the *preparation* stage, people intend to take action soon (within one month), knowing that the change is beneficial to them and is possible to achieve [88, 93, 96]. They have often already made some significant changes in the past year. They have a plan of action, such as visiting health education workshops, obtaining advice from an advisor and purchasing self-help books, or opt for the independent behaviour change approach [87].

People in the *action* stage have made specific, obvious changes in their lifestyles in the last six months [93]. The action can be observed; therefore, the change in behaviour is often equated with it. Action occurs when an individual abandons an unhealthy behaviour, for example ceases smoking, not merely by reducing the number of cigarettes smoked or replacing cigarettes with those having a lower tar and nicotine content [87].

Maintenance is the stage in which people have made certain obvious changes to their lifestyles and strive to avoid a relapse but without using the change processes as often as people in the action stage. The temptation to relapse is lower, and they are more confident that they can continue with their changing [88, 96]. They slowly begin to realize the advantages of behavioural changes [93]. Based on data on temptation and self-efficacy, it has been estimated that maintenance lasts from six months to about five years [87].

The behaviour of subjects in the *termination* stage becomes automatic. Examples are adults who put on their seat belt as soon as they get into the car or those that automatically take their medicines to lower blood pressure every day, at the same time and in the same place [87]. A study of ex-smokers and alcoholics found that less than 20% of people in each group reached the stage of no temptation and complete self-efficacy [87, 97]. The criterion may be too strict or perhaps this stage is the ideal goal for most people. In other areas, such as exercise, consistent use of condoms and weight control, maintained change could be a realistic goal for the temptation to relapse is dominant and powerful. Much less research has been performed regarding the termination stage than for the other stages [87].

3.3.3. Processes of change

The processes of change are covert and disclosed activities that individuals use to transition through the stages (levels) of change. Ten coping strategies that people use to transition through the stages of change [93, 98] are given below, which, based on research, have received the greatest empirical support [87]:

- *Consciousness raising (awareness)* includes increasing awareness of the causes, consequences and treatments of an individual's behavioural problem. Interventions that can increase awareness include response, confrontation, interpretation, therapy with the help of books and media campaigns.
- *Dramatic relief* initially produces a heightened emotional experience, followed by a reduced impact or envisioned relief by implementing an appropriate course of action. Role-playing, grief, personal stories, feedback regarding health risks and mass media campaigns are examples of techniques that can touch people emotionally.
- *Self-reevaluation* combines both cognitive and affective evaluation of the individual's self-esteem, with and without the unhealthy behaviour. It is an individual assessment of ourselves as a passive or active person. Interpretation of values, healthy role models and imagery are techniques which may result in individuals evaluating themselves.
- *Environmental reevaluation* combines both cognitive and affective assessment of how the presence or absence of an individual behaviour affects an individual's social environment. An example is the impact of the behaviour of the individual, for example smoking, on their surroundings. It can also include the awareness that one represents a positive or negative role model to others. Empathy training, documentaries, testimonials and family mediation can lead to such a reassessment.
- *Self-liberation* is the belief that one can change, and the individual is committed to striving in this direction. New Year's resolutions, public testimonials and mass selection can strengthen one's willpower.
- *Helping relationships* require one to increase social opportunities or alternatives, especially for people who are relatively disadvantaged or oppressed. Advocacy, authorization procedures and suitable policies can create greater opportunities for minority health promotion and health promotion among homosexuals and poor people. The same procedures can also be used as an aid in change for all people. Examples of these are non-smoking areas, salad bars in school canteens, and easy access to condoms and other contraceptives.

- *Counterconditioning* requires the individual to learn a healthier mode of behaviour, which can replace problematic behaviour. Strategies for healthier behaviour include release, various arguments, substitutes for nicotine and positive self-statements.
- *Reinforcement management* removes reminders of unhealthy habits and adds signs for healthier alternatives. Avoidance, a new choice of social environment and self-help groups may be incentives that support change and reduce the risk of a relapse.
- *Stimulus control* involves consequences for wrong decisions. Despite the fact that stimulus control involves the application of penalties on persons who are striving for self-change, it relies more on awards than on punishment. The philosophy of the stage model is that it takes place in harmony with the way people themselves naturally change, so here, fortification is primarily emphasized. Procedures for increasing fortification of and the probability that healthy responses will continue are unforeseeable contracts, visible and invisible reinforcement, encouragement and recognition given by groups.
- *Social liberation* combines caring, trust, openness and acceptance, as well as support for a healthy behavioural change. Sources of social support may include the establishment of contacts, therapeutic relationships, consultant calls and a peer system.

3.3.4. Studies that have shown the positive effects of using the transtheoretical model

There have been a number of studies carried out in which the distribution of stages for a precise determination of behaviours with increased risk such as smoking was first established [99, 100, 101, 102, 103, 104]. Researchers were also interested in determining the systematic relationships between the stage the individual was in and the processes of change which they were subjected to [86, 87]. Many intervention studies were also performed to identify their connection with the TTM for smoking cessation, dietary habits, physical activity, stress management, taking of medication, alcohol abuse and use of condoms. TTM has been used in various areas, including kindergartens, at home, in schools, churches, campuses, and in different communities and workplaces. Several studies showing the usefulness of TTM are presented next [87].

In a study conducted in Thailand among pregnant women and women with young children (n = 315), the progression of implementing preventative behaviour in stages for preventing passive smoking was established. They found that knowledge on the effects of exposure to passive smoking of health care professionals had a positive impact on women in the precontemplation stage. For those who are in the action or maintenance stages, practicing preventive behaviours in different situations and learning communication skills as well as effective and appropriate communication with smokers are important [105].

Haakstad et al. [106] used TTM to measure the readiness of pregnant women to become or stay physically active. Healthy pregnant women (n = 467), 32 – 36 weeks pregnant, who responded to the questionnaire on physical activity to assess what stage of TTM they were in participated. The results showed that the acquisition of advice from health professionals can increase the likelihood that pregnant women would fall under higher stages of the change process (stages 4–5), while older age, obesity, poor diet, pelvic pain and urinary incontinence increase the likelihood of poor readiness to change exercise habits (stages 1–3). Despite the fact that many pregnant women were categorized as inactive, these were the ones who displayed a high motivational willingness or intention to increase their level of physical activity. Thus, pregnancy can also be an opportunity to establish long-term habits of physical activity.

A study on adult volunteers (n = 1455) in the USA established a link between body satisfaction and the use of TTM for changing behaviour – physical activity. The results showed a characteristic statistical change in body satisfaction depending on the stage of change. The highest satisfaction that was found was in the final stage and the lowest in the precontemplation stage. Participants with higher body satisfaction are often tempted to leave out physical activity, which was contrary to the initial expectations. Those found to be already in the initial stages were more satisfied with their bodies and mostly remained in the stage in which they were at the beginning because they did not feel the need to change, since nothing regarding their bodies bothered them, and they therefore did not contemplate the benefits of exercise [107].

A research carried out on adult women in Pennsylvania (n = 27) studied whether the use of TTM in strength training programmes had an impact on the likelihood of behavioural change. The use of TTM has shown positive effects in progressing from a lower to a higher stage of change, facilitating decision-making in relation to the advantages and disadvantages of introducing changes and increasing general physical capacity [108].

3.4. Motivation for change

The term "motivation" is used to refer to our reasons for action (what our motives are) and our enthusiasm for doing them (how motivated we are) [109]. Motivation can be internal or external. The concept of internal motivation was developed to explain people's desire to carry out certain activities without external rewards – the motivation for such behaviour was the satisfaction of some internal needs and that the individual feels competent to make their own decisions [110]. Internal motivation is encouraged by three universal human needs, namely the need for autonomy, competence and affiliation. When an individual is free to choose their own activities (autonomy), when they master activities (competence) and when important people support the individual in these endeavours (affiliation), it is highly likely that the individual will carry out the activities with happiness and internal satisfaction. So in order to establish a certain behaviour, internal motivation and self-determination are needed which arise from satisfying the aforementioned needs [109, 110]. An individual who is internally motivated (*intrinsic motivation*; coming from within, like an aspiration to do something due to a desire to be a "better person") does not require a stimulus from the environment and expands their interests and develops and obtains new knowledge; for this individual, the path to the goal is more important than the goal itself [111, 112]. In the case of external motivation (*extrinsic motivation*), it is a fact that people are motivated to make a change if they are rewarded for doing so (e.g. praise, fear, coercion, material goods, beautiful appearance, recognition from the surroundings, fame, acknowledgement). These people are dependent on the opinions of people in their environment and on external stimuli [112, 113].

One of the most famous theories, namely the TTM theory, is strongly related to motivation. This defines the type of motivational stages through which people pass; however, they could also repeat (relapse) unhealthy behaviours [85]. The TTM theory is most commonly used for health education and health promotion, such as for the cessation of smoking, use of condoms, weight loss, drug abuse and stress management [114]. Many psychological theories define motivation as an important behavioural factor. However, it is difficult to identify the various factors that influence motivation, including conscious and unconscious processes, internal and external influences, different beliefs regarding the consequences of one's current behaviour, expected results of the new behaviour and perceptions of social norms [109].

In order to implement a change, the individual must be motivated [31]. Dilts et al. [115] point out that when changing the lifestyle habits of an individual, one must take into account their environments and personality traits, which are defined as behaviour, strategies (skills and abilities), beliefs, values, identity, mission and spirituality.

Most core behavioural change theories include both the individual's motivation and also their confidence. This regards the confidence of the individual that they will be able to implement a change in behaviour, in other words, their confidence in their capabilities. The concept can also be called self-efficacy and represents the basis of models and theories such as the health-belief model and social cognitive theory and that of perceived behavioural control in the theory of planned behaviour [109].

The concepts of confidence and motivation differ from one another, but they are also linked. From the literature, it is evident that motivational factors and self-efficacy are important when designing intentions (i.e. the individual's obligation to carry out a certain behaviour). Intentions express the individual's motivation to achieve a certain objective [31, 109].

It is important that health professionals be familiar with the ways in which individuals who opt for a lifestyle change can be effectively motivated. One such way is motivational interviewing which is suitable for all areas of lifestyle change, especially when the individual already requires treatment [116].

3.4.1. Motivational interviewing

The concept of motivational interviewing was developed by Muller from his experience of treating alcoholism and was first described in 1983 [117]. Motivational interviewing is an advisory technique that increases the individual's motivation to change problematic behaviours [118, 119]. As an advisory technique, it involves strengthening the patient's motivation to change using the following four guiding principles: encouraging the patient's independence, understanding the patient's own motivation, empathic listening and encouraging the patient – giving the patient power [120].

With the aid of motivational interviewing, during the communication process, the health professional can assess the readiness of the patient (client) to change, assist them in entering the next stage of the change process, and direct and guide them through the change process [121, 122, 123]. This is a technique that highlights an individual's ambivalence regarding change and their arguments "for" and "against" change [121, 122, 124, 125]. The advisor in using motivational interviewing helps the individual adopt important life decisions. Ambivalent individuals are characterized by their difficulty to make decisions [121, 122]. Motivational interviewing is particularly useful in helping clients identify current and potential problems and do something about them [126].

The basic assumption in motivational interviewing is that the change will occur if the client is ready for it [127]. The main components of motivational interviewing comprise assessment of the individual's readiness to change, provision of feedback (e.g. in the form of praise, respect and understanding; encouraging the individual during the process of introducing changes), avoidance of resistance, negotiation of goals and strategies, coping with ambivalence, determination of the level of significance of the change and assessment of the individual's confidence in their own ability to change [128].

A major characteristic of motivation interviewing is the patient-oriented manner of counselling, which seeks to change the behaviour of the patient leading them to explore and resolve their ambivalence to changes. Telling individuals what they should do, using persuasion employing logic, arguments, lectures, or provision of advice or solutions are conceptually opposites of motivational interviewing [129]. Motivational interviewing is by no means a technique whereby we manipulate people into doing something they do not want to do! It is a clinical advisory skill that enables people to recognize their own health motives necessary for deciding to change their behaviour. This involves management of more so than prescribing [129, 130]. It is a support action of the advisor who seeks to enhance the inner motivation of the individual so that the change comes from within and not from outside [119].

The most important concepts describing the philosophy of motivational interviewing are participation, respect for the individual's autonomy and elicitation. A collaborative conversation is carried out between the individual and advisor, developed through a collective decision-making process. The basic skills of motivational interviewing comprise therapeutic tools that help build relationships, explore concerns and provide empathy. This includes "open" questions, affirmations, reflective listening and summarization [119, 129, 130]. Authors in the context of communication techniques recommend the use of open questions to aid in determining what the problem means to a person and how they will remedy it. This technique is particularly useful for people who health professionals have previously assessed as "resistant to change" [96]. A major characteristic of open questions is that the individual speaks the majority of the time while the health professional (advisor) poses targeted questions including: What are the disadvantages of your current situation, what are the benefits of change, how optimistic are you about change and what is the purpose of the change [131]? Reflective listening is a communication strategy involving two key steps: seeking to understand the speaker's idea a nd then offering the idea back to the speaker using the listener's own words (without paraphrasing), to confirm the idea has been understood correctly [132].

3.4.2. Studies that have shown the positive effects of using motivational interviewing

Motivational interviewing is a well-known scientific testing method to provide advice to clients and is regarded as a useful intervention strategy for treating problems regarding lifestyle and disease. A systematic review and meta-analysis of randomized controlled studies showed that motivational interviewing in the scientific environment outperforms traditional advice for behavioural problems and illnesses [126]. Motivational interviewing was used and evaluated in relation to alcohol abuse, drug addiction, smoking cessation, weight loss, increase in fruit and vegetable intake [133, 134], adherence to treatments and follow-up, increase in physical activity, and treatment of asthma and diabetes [126, 127]. No research found any negative effects of using motivational interviewing. It has been used by various health care providers, including psychologists, doctors, nurses and midwives [126, 135, 136, 137]. The literature review found motivational interviewing to already be effective after only15 minutes of use and that more than one session increases the possibility of a positive effect on the individual [124, 135, 138, 139, 140, 141].

Over 200 randomized controlled studies showed that motivational interviewing can encourage changes in behaviour in different health care facilities, improve relationships between patients and doctors, and increase the effectiveness of counselling [142] and that it has positive effects on many aspects of health [143]. The impact of the use of motivational interviewing in health was established in a randomized controlled study conducted on patients (n = 146) with low motivation for a healthy lifestyle by the Cardiac Rehabilitation Centre in Hong Kong. They found that motivational interviewing had long-term positive effects because it primarily affects the psychological aspects of the quality of life (motivation, emotional stability, depression, stress management) and eventually also helps improve general well-being and reduce physical pain. It has no direct effect on specific factors such as blood pressure, cholesterol, etc. [144].

3.4.2.1. Discussion

Before the midwife decides on how to implement health education and health promotion, it is important that she knows how to explain what health is, because health can have different meanings for the individual. For some, health may mean the absence of disease and disability, while for others it means adaptability [50]. Health is defined in two ways. The first definition defines health as a positive or "wellness" approach, where it is necessary to look at health as means or ability to do something. The second defines health as a negative approach, in which health is the absence of disease [145]. One should keep in mind that individuals value their health in very different ways; health to some regards the highest value, while others rank health somewhat lower on the scale of values. Ranking of health as the highest on the scale of values by an individual does not mean that they act in accordance with this. This conclusion is also supported by findings that individuals desire to do more for their health even though they believe that they already care greatly for it [3].

Some experts have come to the conclusion that lifestyle and health are closely linked and that in order to achieve the highest possible level of health, behaviour harmful to health should be eliminated (unhealthy lifestyles) [146]. Lifestyle is a way to live one's life story – the creation of an individual, in which a constant interplay between the individual and society plays a major role. Lifestyle is a set of habits and use of goods, space and time by which people define themselves and other people; it is a characteristic of groups but also an individual experience [147]. Lifestyle connected to health regards attitudes and values, especially in terms of behaviour (conduct) in various fields, such as sexual health, regular physical activity, healthy and balanced diet, maintenance of normal body weight, stress management, and the cessation of smoking and consumption of alcohol and illicit drugs. Lifestyle cannot be changed quickly.

It is formed in close interaction with one's living conditions. The literature most frequently mentions a pro-health/healthy lifestyle and a harmful/unhealthy lifestyle. The impact of lifestyle on health in individual socio-economic communities can be an indicator of social problems of particular groups of residents. Harmful health habits are said to be indicators of psychosocial stress, which poorer and less- educated people experience due to relative material deprivation and social and psychological deprivation [148].

In determining the lifestyle of the individual, Croghan [149] says that the need of the individual should be included in dialogues on issues related to lifestyle change, because the resulting data are crucial to the individual's attempt to change. When an individual decides to change, it is necessary to assess their readiness to change and the probability of it occurring in a plan for behaviour change. Black et al. [150] also point out that the approach of the nurse/midwife needs to be caring and, at the same time, provide a positive message. It is important that the nurse/ midwife presents a positive image, makes a good first impression, provides a positive message, is a role model for individuals, is aware of their impact on others, and has sufficient knowledge and skills to deal with the unexpected; this indicates that in the process of health education, we should provide assistance to individuals so that they learn how to prevent health problems and how to follow the doctor's instructions.

Health professionals, doctors, nurses, midwives, physiotherapists, occupational therapists and others, play various roles in implementing health education, which are intertwined and complement and supplement each other. It is particularly important that they know how to transition from one role to another while establishing a relaxing and trusting relationship with the individual. Naidoo and Wills [56] state that the nurse/midwife requires two competences in the role of a health educator, namely education and caring. The first relates mainly to scientific knowledge, while the other regards values. Both are heavily dependent on the educator's personality structure. The midwife acquires scientific knowledge by going through technical and scientific literature. In addition, it is also important, as stated by Thiedke [151], that individuals desire consultation with health professionals who provide them with enough information regarding their medical condition or illness and involve them in decision-making. This can only be done if they have enough knowledge, through continual upgrading and supplementation of their existing knowledge. Black et al. [150] found that health professionals are more involved in health promotion and health education if they believe that they have the appropriate knowledge and skills, time, and the support of the environment and recipients. An additional factor that may affect the success of interventions for health promotion and health education is the credibility of health professionals.

Individuals when receiving information and during the learning process are very attentive to the communication that takes place with the midwife. Communication by the midwife requires self-control and self-organization. This improves the knowledge of individuals and leads to the effective improvement of health. People understand only 50% of what is said in the verbal communication of health professionals, leading to misunderstandings and incomplete understanding of the actual health status of the individual [31]. The hermeneutic phenomeno-logical studies on communication between patients and nurses in general hospitals in Ireland found that if nurses used a patient-oriented approach, evaluated and identified as appropriate in health care organizations, they could communicate well with their patients [131].

In the stage of acquiring data regarding the lifestyle of the individual, the midwife evaluates the former's health literacy, which is crucial for planning the health education process. This is also confirmed by Nutbeam [29, 152] and Peerson and Saunders [153], who consider that if a health- risk behaviour is to be eliminated, the health literacy of the individual must first be assessed, for high health literacy affects not only changes in lifestyle but also changes in social, economic and environmental factors of health.

As mentioned previously, following an assessment of health literacy, the midwife together with the individual plans the change of the latter's unhealthy lifestyle. This can be done by using TTM, which, according to Miller and Rollnick [154], is a comprehensive conceptual model and explains how and why changes occur. TTM according to Prochaska and DiClemente [88] is considered an intervention strategy in the treatment of problems related to lifestyle and disease [126]. The positive effects of using TTM have been researched in numerous randomized controlled studies. Researchers found that TTM from initial studies on smoking quickly spread to behavioural research in the broader field of health and mental health, including studies on alcohol and other substance abuse, anxiety and panic disorders, bullying, delinquency, depression, eating disorders and obesity, diets high in fat, prevention of HIV/AIDS, coping with stress, various medical interventions (e.g. vaccinations), impact on healthy sexual behaviour, mammography and other cancer screening, compliance with the use of various medication, prevention of unintended pregnancies, pregnancy and smoking, inactive lifestyle, sun exposure, etc. Researchers were also interested in determining what the connection with behaviour modification is when it comes to changing multiple risky behaviours [155, 156, 157]. A literature review of numerous meta-analyses concluded that risk factors can be successfully prevented by using TTM [157]. Researchers further found that if individuals changed a single behaviour, such as physical activity, this had a positive effect on another behavioural area such as nutrition [158, 159]. This is especially important when dealing with individuals who require a change in a large number of risky behaviours, which is very frequent. The successful change of one behaviour can effect a change in a second behaviour [159].

The individual transitions through a series of stages during the behavioural change process with their motivation for change being of key importance. We can motivate them by using motivational interviewing, which is regarded as an intervention strategy in the treatment of problems related to lifestyle and disease [126]. This is based on the assumption that people become more committed to what they say themselves or what they have heard from others. This, in fact, gives people the opportunity to express arguments for change (conversations regarding change), which predicts that the behaviour will change [160, 161, 162].

During the behavioural change process, it is very important that midwives and other health professionals be a role model for individuals. Individuals expect midwives and other health professionals to behave in a healthy manner. Black et al. [150] suggest that the health professional be involved in the change process along with the individual, for this will enable the health professional to give recommendations to others, while individuals will be more motivated to change their behaviour if their therapist is their role model.

Personal experience in the change process represents a big challenge for the midwife because it requires skills and knowledge regarding a healthy lifestyle and the manner in which to achieve it. Therefore, it is very important that lifelong education/learning be a priority and commitment for the midwife. It is important that she obtain knowledge and skills through various trainings, seminars, and professional and scientific literature. Researchers [150] found that health professionals are more involved in health promotion and health education if they believe that they have the appropriate knowledge and skills, time, and the support of the environment and recipients. An additional factor that may affect the success of interventions for health promotion is the credibility of health workers.

3.5. Conclusion and recommendations

Health education is a discipline that relies on knowledge of different disciplines such as andragogy, pedagogy, didactics, and psychology and sociology; nevertheless, it remains within the scope of the health profession, drawing on the profession's principles in processes related to both healthy and ill individuals. It can be a daily aid for midwives and other health professionals in the processes of preserving and fortifying health as well as treatment and rehabilitation. With health education, the midwife can influence the individual's behaviour and life habits in a positive way, thus contributing to an improved life, reduced health inequality and improved health of the population. Using the knowledge gained through health education, individuals will be able to understand, clarify their position or create new ones, become acquainted with new values and respect them, and pay attention to their health-related behaviour.

We can find a variety of health behaviours in individuals, which may also be harmful to them, such as unhealthy sexuality, an unbalanced diet, increased body weight, physical inactivity, smoking, stress, etc. In this case, we are talking about an unhealthy lifestyle which the individual with the help of a health care professional (midwife) can successfully eliminate. Individuals behave in a variety of different ways (behaviour); some respond to health care messages that promote the maintenance, enhancement and restoration of health, while others ignore them. Planning models based on behavioural health theories can prove to be of great assistance to midwives in eliminating behaviour which represents health risks. TTM is very frequently used by midwives and assists them in determining which of the six stages of behavioural change an individual is in. It also helps them in creating effective strategies for coping with change and encouraging individuals to transit through the individual stages. Due to the fact that individuals are more or less motivated to change, the midwife can use motivational interviewing to significantly increase the inner motivation of individuals to change their behaviour. When an individual passes through the stages of behaviour change, it is extremely important that they adopt the decision to change themselves and not the midwife. During the change process, the individual should be active in solving their own problems while understanding that the midwife understands them and is committed to the individual's development and progress. The individual is able to take a resolution to overcome their problems if the midwife encourages and helps them only to the extent necessary. The midwife should act as a facilitator and never as a "traditional" teacher where the individual is in a subordinate position. Individuals desire a fair and respectful attitude, the opportunity to converse and active listening on the part of the midwife, adequate time for questions and the ability to cope with their current problems.

We should not forget that the process of health education begins with the selection of a suitable space (room). The room should be bright, airy, spacious, and equipped with the appropriate furniture and teaching aids (posters, models, schemes, various brochures, leaflets, books). No one should bother the midwife in the room during the implementation of health education (no ringing phones or visits by colleagues or other clients). The midwife should focus her attention on the individual the moment they enter the room. The midwife should begin the introductory meeting with a greeting, introduce herself, explain the purpose of the visit and tell the individual that they will obtain information. This should be followed by the setting of objectives, creation of a plan and evaluation of the level of health education. It is important that the midwife is flexible when planning and implementing health education, meaning that she continuously adapts to the individual's needs and expectations. During the teaching process, she should always give the individual written materials (e.g. leaflets, brochures, booklets) which she explains to them in advance, giving them the opportunity to ask additional questions and request explanations. The midwife should record everything that is happening with and to the individual promptly in the documentation earmarked for this purpose.

Author details

Andreja Kvas*

Address all correspondence to: andreja.kvas@zf.uni-lj.si

University of Ljubljana, Faculty of Health Sciences, Nursing Department, Slovenia

References

[1] Zaletel-Kragelj L, Eržen I, Premik M. Introduction to Public Health (in Slovenian). Ljubljana: Faculty of Medicine, Department of Public Health; 2011.

[2] World Health Organization. Health Promotion. Global Conferences on Health Promotion; Geneva: World Health Organization; 2014. http://www.who.int/healthpromotion/conferences/en/ (accessed 10 October 2014).

[3] Kamin T. Health on the Barricades: The Dilemmas of Health Promotion (in Slovenian). Ljubljana: Faculty of Social Sciences; 2004.

[4] Whitelaw S, Baxendale A, Bryce C, MacHardy L, Young I, Witney E. Settings based health promotion: A review. Health Promotion International 2001; 16(4): 339–353.

[5] Cross R. Accident and emergency nurses' attitudes towards health promotion. Journal of Advanced Nursing 2005; 51(5): 474–483.

[6] Maben J, Macleod Clark J. Health promotion: A concept analysis. Journal of Advanced Nursing 1995; 22(6): 1158–1165.

[7] Rash ME. Simulating health promotion in an online environment. Journal of Nursing Education 2008; 47(11): 515–517.

[8] Whitehead D. Health promotion and health education: Advancing the concepts. Journal of Advanced Nursing 2004; 47(3): 311–320.

[9] O'Byrne D. Health Education and Health Promotion: Five Year Plan of Action 1998–2002. Geneva: World Health Organization; 1998.

[10] World Health Organization. Gender and Health: Technical Paper. Women's Health and Development, Family and Reproductive Health. Geneva: World Health Organization; 1998.

[11] Wendt E, Hildingh C, Lidell E, Westerstal A, Baigi A, Marklund B. Young women's sexual health and their views on dialogue with health professionals. Acta Obstetricia et Gynecologica 2007; 86(5): 590–595.

[12] Weeks J. Sexuality. London, New York: Routledge; 1986.

[13] Giddens A. The Transformation of Intimacy: Sexuality, Love and Eroticism in Modern Societies. Cambridge: Polity Press, University of Calgary; 1992.

[14] Getzfeld AR. Essentials of Abnormal Psychology. New York: John Wiley & Sons Inc. ; 2006.

[15] World Health Organization. Defining Sexual Health: Report of a Technical Consultation on Sexual Health. Geneva: World Health Organization; 2006.

[16] Hellström O. Dialogue medicine: A health-liberating attitude in general practice. Patient Education and Counseling 1998;/35(3):/221–231.

[17] Clark PG. Toward a transtheoretical model of interprofessional education: Stages, processes and forces supporting institutional change. Journal of Interprofessional Care 2013; 27(1): 43–49.

[18] Wendt E, Hildingh C, Lidell E, Westerstahl, A, Baigi A, Marklund B. Young women's sexual health and their views on dialogue with health professionals. Acta Obstetricia et Gynecologica Scandinavica 2007; 86(5): 590–595.

[19] Firestone RW, Firestone LA, Catlett J. What is healthy sexuality? In: Sex & Love in Intimate Relationship. Washington, DC: American Psychological Association ; 2006. p. 11–21.

[20] Davis TC, Crouch MA, Long SW, et al. Rapid assessment of literacy levels of adult primary care patients. Family Medicine1991; 23(6): 433–435.

[21] Parker RM, Baker DW, Williams MC, Nurss JR. The test of functional HEALTH literacy in adults: A new instrument for measuring patients' literacy skills. Journal of General Internal Medicine 1995; 10(10): 537–541.

[22] Diamond JJ. Development of a reliable and construct valid measure of nutritional literacy in adults. Nutrition Journal 2007; 6: 5.

[23] Nath CR, Sylvester ST, Yasek V, Gunel E. Development and validation of a literacy assessment tool for persons with diabetes. Diabetes Education 2001; 27(6): 857–864.

[24] Levasseur M, Carrier L. Do rehabilitation professionals need to consider their clients' health literacy for effective practice? Clinical Rehabilitation 2010; 24(8): 756–765.

[25] Baker D, Parker R, Williams M, Clark W. Health literacy and the risk of hospital admissions. Journal of General Internal Medicine 1998; 13(12): 791–798.

[26] Baker DW, Gazmararian JA, Williams MV, Scott T, Parker RM, Green D, et al. Functional health literacy and the risk of hospital admission among medicare managed care en rollees. American Journal Public Health 2002; 92(8): 1278–1283.

[27] Kickbusch I. Health literacy: Addressing the health and education divide. Health Promotion International 2001; 16(3): 289–297.

[28] Kickbusch I, Wait S, Maag D. Navigating Health: The Role of Health Literacy. London: International Longevity Centre – UK; 2008. www.ilcuk.org.uk/files/pdf_pdf_3.pdf (accessed 15 November 2014).

[29] Nutbeam D. Health literacy as a public goal: A challenge for contemporary health education and communication strategies into the 21st century. Health Promotion International 2000; 15(3): 259–267.

[30] Van Servellen G. Communication Skills for the Health Care Professional: Concepts, Practice and Evidence, 2 nd edn. Sudbury: Jones and Barlett; 2009.

[31] DeWalt DA, Callahan LF, Hawk VH, Bruckson KA, Hink A. Health literacy universal precautions. Toolkit AHRQ Publication; 2010. http://nchealthliteracy.org/toolkit/toolkit_w_appendix.pdf (accessed 15 November 2014).

[32] Kickbusch I, Maag D. International encyclopedia of public health. In: Heggenhougen K, Quah S, eds. International Encyclopedia of Public Health. San Diego: Academic Press; 2008. p. 204–211.

[33] Vanderhoff M. Patient education and health literacy. Magazine of Physical Therapy 2005; 13: 42–46.

[34] Mancuso JM. Health literacy: A concept/dimensional analysis. Nursing & Health Sciences 2008; 10(3): 248–255.

[35] Howard D H, Gazmararian J, Parker RM. The impact of low health literacy on the medical costs of medicare managed care enrollees. American Journal of Medicine 2005; 118(4): 371–377.

[36] Sudore RL, Yaffe K, Satterfield S, Harris TB, Mehta KM, Simonsick EM, et al. Limited literacy and mortality in the elderly. Journal of General Internal Medicine 2006; 21(8): 806–812.

[37] Kutner M, Greenberg E, Baer J. National Assessment of Adult Literacy (NAAL). A first look at the literacy of America's adults in the 21st century. http://nces.ed.gov/naal (accessed 15 November 2014).

[38] Kripalani S, Jacobson JA, Mugalla IC, Cawthon CR, Niesner KJ, Vaccarino V. Health literacy and the quality of physician-patient communication during hospitalization. Journal of Hospital Medicine 2010; 5(5): 269–275.

[39] Katz MG, Jacobson TA, Veledar E, Kripalani S. Patient literacy and question asking behavior in the medical encounter: A mixed-methods analysis. Journal of General Internal Medicine 2007; 22(6): 782–786.

[40] Davis TC, Wolf MS, Bass PF, III, et al. Literacy and misunderstanding prescription-drug labels. Annals of Internal Medicine 2006; 145(12): 887–894.

[41] Williams MV, Baker DW, Parker RM, Nurss JR. Relationship of functional health literacy to patients' knowledge of their chronic disease: A study of patients with hypertension and diabetes. Archives of Internal Medicine 1998; 158(2): 166–172.

[42] Cavanaugh KL, Wingard RL, Hakim RM, Eden S, Shintani A, Wallston A, Huizinga MM, Elasy TA, Rothman RL, Ikizler TA. Low health literacy associates with increased mortality in ESRD. Journal of American Society Nephrology 2010; 21(11): 1979–1985.

[43] Wilhelmova R, Hruba D, Vesela L. Key determinants influencing the health literacy of pregnant women in the Czech republic. Journal of Public Health 2015; 54(1): 27–36.

[44] Kickbusch IS. Health literacy: Addressing the health and education divide. Health Promotion International 2001; 16(3): 289–297.

[45] World Health Organization. Health Promotion Glossary. Geneva: World Health Organization; 1998.

[46] Suhrcke M, de Paz Nieves C. The impact of health and health behaviours on educational outcomes in highincome countries: A review of the evidence. Copenhagen: WHO Regional Office for Europe; 2011.

[47] World Health Organization. Milestones in Health Promotion Statements from Global Conference. Geneva: World Health Organization; 2009.

[48] Sussex F, Herne D, Scourfield P. Advanced Health and Social Care for NVQ Level 4 and Foundation Degree. Ashford Colour Press Ltd.; 2008.

[49] World Health Organisation. The Ottawa Charter for Health Promotion. Geneva: World Health Organization; 1986. http://www.who.int/healthpromotion/conferences/previous/ottawa/en/ (accessed 15 November 2014).

[50] Kiger A. Teaching for Health, 3rd edn. Edinburgh: Churchill Livingstone; 2004.

[51] World Health Organization. World Health Statistics. Geneva: World Health Organization; 2012. http://apps.who.int/iris/bitstream/10665/44844/1/9789241564441_eng.pdf (accessed 20 November 2014).

[52] World Health Organization. Health Education: Theoretical Concepts, Effective Strategies and Core Competencies: A Foundation Document to Guide Capacity Development of Health Educators. Regional Office for the Eastern Mediterranean, World Health Organization; 2012.

[53] Green L, Kreuter M. Health Promotion Planning: An Educational and Environmental Approach. Palo Alto : Mayfield Publishing; 1991.

[54] Sluijs EM, Knibbe JJ. Patient compliance with exercises: Different theoretical approaches to short-term and long-term compliance. Patient Education Counseling 1991; 17: 191–204.

[55] Sluijs EM, van der Zee J, Kok GJ. Differences between physical therapists in attention paid to patient education. Physical Theory & Practice 1993; 9: 103–107.

[56] Naidoo J, Wills J. Foundations for Health Promotion, 3rd edn. Edinburgh : Elsevier; 2009.

[57] Glanz K, Rimer BK, Viswanath K. The scope of health behavior and health education. In: Glanz K, Rimer BK, Viswanath K, eds. Health Behavior and Health Education: Theory, Research, and Practice, 4th edn. San Francisco : Jossey-Bass; 2008. p. 3–22.

[58] Piper BS, Brown BA. The theory and practice of health education applied to nursing: Abi-polar approach. Journal of Advanced Nursing 1998; 27(2): 383–389.

[59] Miller PM, Graves KD. Behavioral medicine in the prevention and treatment of cardiovascular disease. Behavior Modification 2003; 27(1): 3–25.

[60] McCabe C, Timmins F. Communication Skills for Nurse Practice. New York: Palgrave Macmillan; 2006.

[61] Caris-Verhallen W, Timmermans L, van Dulmen S. Observation of nurse–patient interaction in oncology: Review of assessment instruments. Patient Education and Counseling 2004; 54(3): 307–320.

[62] Fakhr-Movahedi A, Salsali M, Negharandeh R, Rahnavard Z. A qualitative content analysis of nurse–patient communication in Iranian nursing. International Nursing Review 2011; 58(2): 171–180.

[63] Thomas RK. Health Communication. New York: Springer Science and Business Media Inc; 2006.

[64] Hagerty BM, Patusky KL. Reconceptualizing the nurse–patient relationship. Journal of Nursing Scholarship 2003; 35(2): 145–150.

[65] Markides M. The importance of good communication between patient and health professionals. Journal of Pediatric Hematology Oncology 2011; 33(Supp 2): S123–S125.

[66] Roberts L, Bucksey SJ. Communicating with patients: What happens in practice? Journal of Physical Therapy 2007; 87(5): 586–594.

[67] Hartley P. Interpersonal Communication. London: Routledge; 1993.

[68] Klisiari A, Gaki A. The concept of communication between nurse and patient in the catheterization laboratory. Hospital Chronicles 2012; 7(1): 26–30.

[69] Charlton CR, Dearing KS, Berry JA, Johnson MJ. Nurse practitioners' communication styles and their impact on patient outcomes: An integrated literature review. Journal of the American Academy of Nurse Practitioners 2008; 20(7): 382–388.

[70] Putnam LL. Shifting voices, oppositional discourse, and new visions for communication. Journal of Communication 2001; 51(1): 38–51.

[71] Gamble M, Gamble TK. Communication Works. Boston: McGraw-Hill College; 2002.

[72] Kinesy Gomana C. The Nonverbal Advantage. San Francisco : Berrett-Koechler Publications, Inc.; 2008.

[73] Rungapadiachy DM. Self-Awareness in Health Care: Engaging in Helping Relationships. Palgrave Macmillan; 2008.

[74] Manojlovich M, Antonakos CL, Ronis DL. Intensive care unites communication between nurses and physicians and patient's outcomes. American Journal of Critical Care 2009; 18(1): 21–30.

[75] Small B. What About Me, What Do I Want? Oxford: Trafford Publishing; 2010.

[76] Kilkus SP. Assertiveness among professional nurses. Journal of Advanced Nursing 1993; 18(8): 1324–1330.

[77] Platt FW, Platt CM. Empathy: A miracle or nothing at all? Journal of Clinical Outcome Management 1998; 5: 30–33.

[78] Champion VL, Sugg Skinner C. The health belief model. In: Glanz K, Rimer BK, Viswanath K, eds. Health Behavior and Health Education: Theory, Research, and Practice, 4th edn. San Francisco : Jossey-Bass; 2008. p. 46–65.

[79] Montano DE, Kasprzyk D. Theory of reasoned action, theory of planned behaviour, and the integrated behavioural model. In: Glanz K, Rimer BK, Viswanath K, eds.

Health Behavior and Health Education: Theory, Research, and Practice, 4th edn. San Francisco : Jossey-Bass; 2008. p. 68–96.

[80] Ben Natan M, Beyil V, Neta O. Nurse's perception of the quality of care they provide to hospitalized drug addicts: Testing the theory of reasoned action. International Journal of Nursing Practice 2009; 15(6): 566–573.

[81] Anderson AG, Lavalee D. Applying the theories of reasoned action and planned behavior to athlete training adherence behavior. International Association of Applied Psychology 2008; 57(2): 304–312.

[82] World Health Organization. List of Basic Terms. Health Promotion Glossary. Geneva: World Health Organization; 1998. p. 4.

[83] Weinstein ND, Sandman PM, Blalock SJ. The precaution adoption process model. In: Glanz K, Rimer BK, Viswanath K, eds. Health Behavior and Health Education: Theory, Research, and Practice, 4th edn. San Francisco : Jossey-Bass; 2008. p. 124–147.

[84] De Vet E, De Nooijer J, Oenema A, De Vries NK, Brug J. Predictors of stage transitions in the precaution adoption process model. American Journal of Health Promotion 2008; 22(4): 282–290.

[85] Prochaska JO, DiClemente CC. Stages and processes of selfchange of smoking: Toward an integrative model of change. Journal of Consult Clinical Psychology 1983; 51(3): 390–395.

[86] Prochaska JO, DiClemente CC, Norcross JC. In search of how people change. Applications to addictive behaviors. American Psychology1992; 47(9): 1102–1114.

[87] Prochaska JO, Redding CA, Evers KE. The transtheoretical model and stages of change. In: Glanz K, Rimer BK, Viswanath K, eds. Health Behavior and Health Education: Theory, Research, and Practice, 4th edn. San Francisco : Jossey-Bass; 2008. p. 98–121.

[88] Prochaska JO, DiClemente CC. The Transtheoretical Approach: Crossing Traditional Boundaries of Change. Homewood : Dorsey Press; 1984.

[89] DiClemente CC, Prochaska JO. Self change and therapy change of smoking behavior. A comparison of processes of change in cessation and maintenance. Addictive Behavior 1982; 7(2): 133–142.

[90] Prochaska JO, DiClemente CC, Norcross JC. In search of how people change: Applications to addictive behaviors. American Psychology 1992; 47(9): 1102–1114.

[91] DiClemente CC. Changing addictive behaviors: A process perspective. Current Directions Psychological Sciences 1993; 2(4): 101–106.

[92] Prochaska JO. Moving beyond the transtheoretical model. Addiction 2006; 101(6): 768–774.

[93] Prochaska JO, Redding CA, Harlow LL, Rossi JS, Velicer WF. The transtheoretical model of change and HIV prevention: A review. Health Education Quarterly 1994; 21(4): 471–486.

[94] Armitage CJ. Can variables from the transtheoretical model predict dietary change? Journal of Behavioral Medicine 2010; 33(4): 264–273.

[95] Dempsey AR, Johnsonand SS, Westhoff CL. Predicting oral contraceptive continuation using the transtheoretical model of health behavior change. Perspectives on Sexual and Reproductive Health 2011; 43(1): 23–29.

[96] Percival J. Promoting health: Making every contact count. Nursing Standard 2014; 28(29): 37–41.

[97] Snow MG, Prochaska JO, Rossi JS. Stages of change for smoking cessation among former problem drinkers: A cross-sectional analysis. Journal of Substance Abuse 1992; 4(2): 107–116.

[98] Sanders R, Burke K. The "hidden" technology of effective parent consultation: A guided participation model for promoting change in families. Journal of Child and Family Studies 2014; 23: 1289–1297.

[99] Velicer WF, Fava JL, Prochaska JO, Abrams DB, Emmons KM, Pierce JP. Distribution of smokers by stage in three representative samples. Preventive Medicine 1995; 24(4): 401–411.

[100] Etter JF, Perneger TV, Ronchi A. Distributions of smokers by stage: International comparison and association with smoking prevalence. Preventive Medicine 1997; 26(4): 580–585.

[101] Yasin SM, Retneswari M, Moy FM, Taib KM, Isahak M, Koh D. Testing the transtheoretical model in predicting smoking relapse among Malaysian adult smokers receiving assistance in quitting. Asian Pacific Journal of Cancer Prevention 2013; 14(4): 2317–2323.

[102] Campbell S, Bohanna I, Swinbourne A, et al. Stages of change, smoking behaviour and readiness to quit in a large sample of indigenous Australians living in eight remote North Queensland communities. International Journal of Environmental Research and Public Health 2013; 10(4): 1562–1571.

[103] Prochaska J, Velicer W, Fava J, et al. Evaluating a population-based recruitment approach and a stage-based expert system intervention for smoking cessation. Addictive Behaviors 2001; 26(4): 583–602.

[104] Huang CM, Wu HL, Huang SH, et al. Transtheoretical model-based passive smoking prevention programme among pregnant women and mothers of young children. European of Journal Public Health 2013; 23(5): 777–782.

[105] Huang CM, Guo JL, Wu HL, Chien LY. Stage of adoption for preventive behaviour against passive smoking among pregnant women and women with young children in Taiwan. Journal of Clinical Nursing 2011; 20(23–24): 3331–3338.

[106] Hagen Haakstad LA, Voldner N, Bø K. Stages of change model for participation in physical activity during pregnancy. Journal of Pregnancy 2013; 167(1): 1–7.

[107] Johnson P, Fallon EA, Harris BS, Burton B. Body satisfaction is associated with transtheoretical model constructs for physical activity behaviour change. Body Image 2013; 10(2): 163–174.

[108] Fetherman DI, Hakim RM, Sanko JP. A pilot study on the application of the transtheoretical model during strength training in older women. Journal of Women & Aging 2011; 23(1): 58–76.

[109] Dixon A. Motivation and Confidence: What Does It Take to Change Behaviour? London: The King's Found; 2008.

[110] Deci EL, Ryan RM. The "what" and "why" of goal pursuits: Human needs and the self determination of behaviour. Psychological Inquiry 2000; 11(4): 227–268.

[111] Ryan RM, Deci EL. Self-determination theory and the facilitation of intrinsic motivation, social development, and well-being. American Psychologist 2000; 55(1): 68–78.

[112] Ellis C. Motivational interviewing: Fostering behavioral change in older clients. CSA Journal 2014; 58: 28–31.

[113] Wigfield A, Guthrie JT, Tonks S, Perencevich, KC. Children's motivation for reading: Domain specificity and instructional influences. Journal of Educational Research 2004; 97(6): 299–309.

[114] West R. Time for a change: Putting the transtheoretical (stages of change) model to rest. Addiction 2005; 100(8): 1036–1039.

[115] Dilts RB, Deering A, Russell J. Leadership cults and cultures. Leader to Leader 2003; 28(2): 31–38.

[116] Marquardt P, Vezeau T. Use of motivational interviewing to facilitate behavioral changes. The American Journal for Nurse Practitioners 2007; 11(8): 21–24, 27–31.

[117] Miller WR. Motivational interviewing with problem drinkers. Behavioural Psychotherapy 1983; 11(2): 147–172.

[118] Rollnick S, Miller WR. What is motivational interviewing? Behavioural and Cognitive Psychotherapy 1995; 23(4): 325–334.

[119] Miller WR, Rollnick S. Motivational Interviewing, Preparing People to Change Addictive Behavior. New York: The Guildford Press; 2002.

[120] Hall K, Gibbie T, Lubman DI. Motivational interviewing techniques. Facilitating behaviour change in the general practice setting. Australian Family Physician 2012; 41(9): 660–667.

[121] Britt E, Hudson SM, Blampied NM. Motivational interviewing in health settings: A review. Patient Education Consulting 2004; 53(2): 147–155.

[122] Gual A, Anderson P, Segura L, Colom J. Alcohol and Primary Health Care: Training Program on Identification and Brief Interventions. Barcelona: Department of Health of the Government of Catalonia; 2005.

[123] Österlund Efraimsson E, Fossum B, Ehrenberg A, Larsson K, Klang K. Use of motivational interviewing in smoking cessation at nurse-led chronic obstructive pulmonary disease clinics. Journal of Advanced Nursing 2011; 8(4): 767–782.

[124] Dunn C, Deroo L, Rivara FP. The use of brief interventions adapted from motivational interviewing across behavioral domains: A systematic review. Addiction 2001; 96(12): 1725–1742.

[125] Resnicow K, Dilkorio C, Soet JE, Borreli B, Hecht J. Motivational interviewing in health promotion: It sounds like something in changing. Health Psychology 2002; 21(5): 444–451.

[126] Rubak S, Sandbæk A, Lauritzen T, Christensen B. Motivational interviewing: A systematic review and meta-analysis. B ritish Journal of General Practice 2005; 55(513): 305–312.

[127] Duran LS. Motivating health: Strategies for the nurse practitioner. Journal of the American Association of Nurse Practitioners 2003; 15(5): 200–205.

[128] Emmons KM, Rollnick S. Motivational interviewing in health care settings: Opportunities and limitations. American Journal of Preventive Medicine 2001; 20(1): 68–74.

[129] Rollnick S, Miller WR, Butler CC. Motivational Interviewing in Health Care: Helping Patients Change Behavior. New York, London: The Guilford Press; 2008.

[130] Rosengren DB. Building Motivational Interviewing Skills (Practitioner Workbook). New York, London: The Guilford Press; 2009.

[131] McCabe C. Nurse–patient communication: An exploration of patients' experiences. Journal of Clinical Nursing 2004; 13(1): 41–49.

[132] Listening ear. What is reflective listening? http://www.listeningearmerseyside.org.uk/information/what-is-reflective-listening (accessed 20 November 2014).

[133] Resnicow K, Jackson A, Want T, De A, McCarty F, Dudley W. A motivational interviewing intervention to increase fruit and vegetable intake through black churches: Results of the eat for life trial. American Journal of Public Health 2001; 91(10): 1686–1693.

[134] Knight KM, McGowan L, Dickens C, Bundy C. A systematic review of motivational interviewing in physical health care settings. British Journal of Health Psychology 2006; 11(2): 319–332.

[135] Berg-Smith SM, Stevens VJ, Brown KM, et al. A brief motivational intervention to improve dietary adherence in adolescents. The Dietary Intervention Study in Children (DISC) Research Group. Health Education Research 1999; 14(3): 399–410.

[136] Tappin DM, Lumsden MA, McIntyre D, et al. A pilot study to establish a randomised trial methodology to test the efficacy of a behavioural intervention. Health Education Research 2000; 15(4): 491–502.

[137] Dilorio C, Resnicow K, McDonnell M, et al. Using motivational interviewing to promote adherence to antiretroviral medications: A pilot study. Journal of the Association of Nurses in AIDS Care 2003; 14(2): 52–62.

[138] Fleming MF, Manwell LB, Barry KL, et al. Brief physician advice for alcohol problems in older adults: A randomised community based trial. Journal of Family Practice 1999; 48(5): 378–384.

[139] Harland J, White M, Drinkwater C, et al. The Newcastle exercise project: A randomised controlled trial of methods to promote physical activity in primary care. BMJ 1999; 319(7213): 828–832.

[140] Rosal MC, Ockene JK, Ma Y, et al. Coronary artery smoking intervention study (CASIS): 5-year follow-up. Journal of Health Psychology 1998; 17(5): 476–478.

[141] Pinto BM, Lynn H, Marcus BH, et al. Physician-based activity counseling: Intervention effects on mediators of motivational readiness for physical activity. Annals of Behavioral Medicine 2001; 23(1): 2–10.

[142] Miller WR, Rose GS. Motivational interviewing in relational context. American Psychologist 2010; 65(4): 298–299.

[143] Miller WR, Rollnick S. Meeting in the middle: Motivational interviewing and self-determination theory. International Journal of Behavioral Nutrition and Physical Activity 2012; 9: 2.

[144] Ying Chair S, Wai-Chi Chan S, Thompson DR, Leung KP, Ka-Chiu Ng S, Chow Choi K. Long-term effect of motivational interviewing on clinical and psychological out comes and health-related quality of life in cardiac rehabilitation patients with poor motivation in Hong Kong: A randomized controlled trial. Clinical Rehabilitation 2013; 27(12): 1107–1117.

[145] Wills J. The role of the nurse in promoting health. In: Wills J, ed. Promoting Health: Vital Notes for Nurses. Oxford : Blackwell Publishing; 2007. p. 1–10.

[146] Tones K, Green I. Health Promotion: Planning and Strategies. London, Thousand Oaks: Sage ; 2004.

[147] Chaney D. Lifestyles. London: Routledge; 1996.

[148] Wilkinson RG. Wilkinson income, inequality and social cohesion. American Journal of Public Health 1997; 87(1): 104–106.

[149] Croghan E. Supporting vulnerable groups during behaviour change. Nursing Standard 2005; 19(36): 48–49.

[150] Black B, Marcous BC, Stiller C, Qu X, Gellish R. Personal health behaviors and role-modeling attitudes of physical therapists and physical therapists students: A cross-sectional study. Physical Therapists 2012; 92(11): 1419–1436.

[151] Thiedke CC. What do we really know about patient satisfaction? Family Practice Management 2007; 14(1): 33–36.

[152] Nutbeam D. The evolving concept of health literacy. Social Science & Medicine 2008; 67(12): 2072–2078.

[153] Peerson A, Saunders M. Health literacy revisited: What do we mean and why does it matter? Health Promotion International 2009; 24(3): 285–296.

[154] Miller WR, Rollnick S. Ten things that motivational interviewing is not. Behavioural and Cognitive Psychotherapy 2009; 37(2): 129–140.

[155] Hall KL, Rossi JS. Meta-analytic examination of the strong and weak principles across 48 health behaviors. Preventive Medicine 2008; 46: 266–274.

[156] Noar SM, Chabot M, Zimmerman RS. Applying health behavior theory to multiple behavior change: Considerations and approaches. Preventive Medicine 2008; 46(3): 275–280.

[157] Johnson BT, Scott-Sheldon AJ, Carey MP. Meta- synthesis of health behavior change meta-analyses. American Journal of Public Health 2010; 100(11): 2193–2198.

[158] French SA, Hennrikus DJ, Jeffery RW. Smoking status, dietary intake, and physical activity in a sample of working adults. Health Psychology 1996; 15(6): 448–454.

[159] Lippke S, Nigg CR, Maddock JE. Health-promoting and health-risk behaviors: Theory-driven analyses of multiple health behavior change in three international samples. International Journal Behavioral Medicine 2012; 19(1): 1–13.

[160] Gaume J, Gmel G, Daeppen JB. Brief alcohol interventions: Do counsellors' and patients' communication characteristics predict change? Alcohol and Alcoholism 2008, 43: 62–69.

[161] van Keulen HM, Mesters I, Ausems M, van Breukelen G, Campbell M, Resnicow K, Brug J, de Vries H. Tailored print communication and telephone motivational interviewing are equally successful in improving multiple lifestyle behaviors in a randomized controlled trial. Annals of Behavioral Medicine 2011; 41: 104–118.

[162] Apodaca TR, Longabaugh R. Mechanisms of change in motivational interviewing: A review and preliminary evaluation of the evidence. Addiction 2009, 104: 705–715.

Chapter 4

Midwifery Students' Perception of Intimate Touch in Clinical Practice

Tita Stanek Zidarič and Metka Skubic

Additional information is available at the end of the chapter

http://dx.doi.org/10.5772/60499

1. Introduction

The term 'intimacy' and 'intimate' from the Latin words *intimus* (innermost) and *intimare* (to make the innermost known) can be used to refer to feelings, to verbal and nonverbal communication processes, to behaviours, to people's arrangements in space, to personality traits, to sexual activities, and to kinds of long-term relationships [1].

In midwifery, touch has many purposes, meanings, and enactments. Some forms of touch do not cross the boundaries of the culturally accepted, while on some occasions, intimate physical touch must be employed in order to provide necessary care. Such touch involves inspection of, and possible physical contact with, those parts of the body whose exposure can cause embarrassment to either the woman, her partner, or the midwife.

Midwifery students who are still in the process of learning may be seen as a special and vulnerable population because in clinical settings, they might feel as outsiders, left alone to tend to their own learning needs, inexperienced in midwifery care, and unsure of their rights; alongside, as young people, they are often still struggling with their own sexual identity, orientation, and sexuality in general. At the same time, it is expected that as midwifery students in clinical practice, they will maintain clear sexual boundaries at all times towards the people for whom they provide care.

2. Literature review

Intimacy usually occurs between two people who influence each other's feelings and behaviour [1]. Pregnancy and childbirth have the potential for being intimate and emotionally charged experiences for all involved [2]. The model of intimacy as shown in Figure 1 shows the comprehensive conceptualization of intimacy that encompasses individual, interactional and relationship qualities [3].

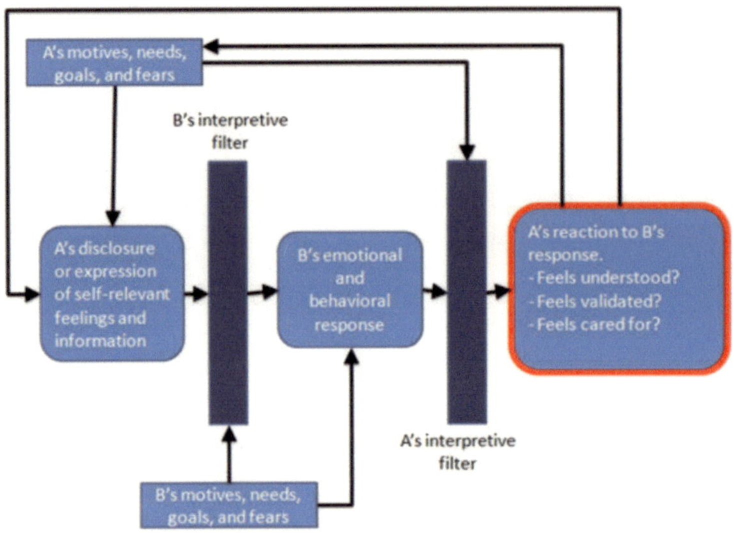

Figure 1. The model of intimacy [1]

The majority of midwifery work involves intimate knowledge of another's body, which normally includes physical contact. Nevertheless, according to [2], contemporary midwifery work is much broader and has several key features:

- Changes in the organization of care, with an emphasis on continuity and the potential increase in the emotional aspect of workMidwives often work in situations where there is a high level of expressed emotionMidwifery work is intimate and involves acknowledgement of sexuality
- Midwives often work with women who are experiencing intense painThe division of labour within maternity care results in additional emotion management.

In the literature, various terms have been used to describe intimate touch. Intimate physical touch is defined as involving 'inspection of, and possible physical contact with those parts of the body whose exposure can cause embarrassment to either the patient or the midwife' [4]. O' Lynn and Krautscheid [5] went into details and defined intimate touch as oriented touch to areas of a patient's body – genitalia, buttocks, perineum, inner thighs, lower abdomen and breasts, as well as other areas, depending upon the patient, nurse or midwife, that may produce feelings of discomfort, anxiety or fear. Women, during pregnancy, birth and postpartum, are often compelled in situations when several different health professionals, consciously or unawares, invade their intimate and personal sphere. Procedures like vaginal and rectal examinations, pubic shaving, enemas and breast palpations that are part of midwifery care can be a brutal invasion in a woman's personal and intimate space if not performed tactfully.

Midwives are dealing with healthy women experiencing a normal life event, but there is evidence from the literature that, for some women at least, giving birth is a sexual experience. All clinical settings, especially the labour ward, are an important and challenging learning area for midwifery students because it is where the students learn in authentic complex situations and in intimate situations [6]. It is crucial to realize that health care professionals need to restore the sense of meaning and stop sleep walking through the professional world. They need to recognize that there is a choice of how to behave and choose excellence over ambivalence in every interaction [7].

Many midwifery students enter midwifery with a sense of awe and wonder, searching for meaning in their lives. Every one of them needs to be encouraged to engage with the powerful search for sense of meaning which brought them to midwifery study [7]. Midwifery practice is an integral part of midwifery education, in which clinical mentors play an important role. Mentors' attitudes, experience and knowledge are influences [8]. Therefore, midwives need to stop sleepwalking through their professional life, wake up and recognize that within every interaction, there is a choice of how to behave and an option to choose excellence over ambivalence [7]. The fact is that clinical mentors influence student midwives while they are on clinical practice and that quality care is more than a set of processes. As Nettleton and Brail [9] pointed out, considerable attention has been given to the benefits of mentorship, but equally, poor mentorship can bring long- lasting consequences for those being mentored. Students who are generally novices in age, social maturity and social responsibility struggle to take on the professional responsibility of providing intimate care to strangers [10]. As Walker and Davis [11] found out, the role of mentors who teach and work with midwifery students on the topic of sexual health is very important, as they help them give confidence when working in this area.

3. Methodology

In this chapter, the study aim and the research question are presented. The research methodologies, specifically qualitative methodology and grounded theory, are described and discussed. This chapter also discusses the methods of study used to investigate the research question. The main ethical considerations are discussed. A description of the selection of participants is provided, and a discussion of the data collection follows. Finally, a summary is presented about the process of data collection, management and analysis.

3.1. Study aim

The process of this research started with identification of the research problem and consequently forming the research question that demarcates the phenomenon to be studied. The primary focus of this research and at the same time the research question of this study therefore is: What are midwifery students' perceptions of intimate touch in clinical practice?

- The aim of this study isTo explore the concepts of midwifery students' perception and experience of intimacyTo capture the students' most typical experiences of intimate touch in clinical practice

3.2. Qualitative methodology

Qualitative methodology guided this research study and therefore formed the basis for the research procedures and strategies. The main attraction of this perspective is that it is person centred and holistic, and, as Rees [12] describes, it concentrates on an individual's perceptions, experiences and personal insights. Furthermore, it attempts to encourage people to express their perceptions of situations or feelings in their own words [12].

3.3. The grounded theory approach

For the purpose of this study, it seemed the most appropriate to adopt the grounded theory approach to close the gap in knowledge about the midwifery student's perception on intimate touch in clinical practice. According to Straus and Corbin [13], grounded theory is a creative process that facilitates the development of a new theory and therefore is an appropriate approach to use when there is a lack of knowledge about a topic. Understanding how midwifery students interact and the factors that influence their behaviour is an important aspect of midwifery care. Furthermore, as Hall et al. [14] pointed out, grounded theory is ideal for capturing the complexity of midwives' and midwifery students' therapeutic exchanges with expectant mothers.

Grounded theory was originally developed by Glaser and Strauss in the 1960s, and it means to make possible the 'systematic discovery of theory from the data of social research' [15]. Strauss and Corbin [13] showed that the purpose of using a grounded theory approach is to develop a theory about phenomena of interest that is faithful to, and illuminates, the area under study.

As Morse [16] pointed out, grounded theory is an important qualitative method which makes major contributions to nursing and therefore also midwifery research. This method offers a systematic approach through the clarification of varied responses and therefore focuses on the social meaning people attach to the world around them.

In grounded theory, the researcher drives a general, abstract theory of a process, action or interaction grounded in the views of participants [17]; therefore, it is important to understand, as also Douglas [18] pointed out, that grounded theory acknowledges the role of the researcher as part of the research but also demands from the researcher to interfere as minimally as possible.

3.4. Ethical considerations

Every aspect of this research study was guided by ethical research standards which are informed consent, confidentiality and anonymity, voluntary participation and the right to withdraw [19].

3.4.1. Informed consent and voluntary participation

In the current study, prior to informed consent being obtained, verbal and written explanations were given to participants regarding the study. This was done when the researchers presented the study to the potential participants. The researchers spoke about the purpose of the study, the procedures and the conditions of consent as well as answered questions. The researchers also spoke about how confidentiality or anonymity for the participant will be ensured. The information sheet was given after the presentation to all students that attended the presentation. Those that showed interest in participating were given a gap of 48 hours between receiving the information and consenting. Two days after the presentation, the researcher got in touch (personally) with the interested participants to find out if they had decided to participate in the study. All 13 students who decided that they wished to participate were given a consent form to sign.

Informed consent is important, as it allows participants to make an informed and voluntary choice to participate or refuse to participate [20]. As Holloway [21] pointed out, the process of informed consent is based firmly within the principle of respect for autonomy and means that participation is voluntary. The participants were made clear that the consent in qualitative research, as Holloway and Wheeler [22] pointed out, is an ongoing process and if they decided to withdraw their consent at any stage during the study, either before or during the interviews, they were free to do so. It was clearly expressed in the written and verbal details that no reason or explanations were required if participants chose to withdraw from the study. However, none of the participants withdrew from participating in the study.

3.4.2. Anonymity and confidentiality

Bluff (2004) [23] points out that ethical issues of anonymity and confidentiality are somewhat unique with grounded theory research, especially when the sample size is small, as in the current study. Furthermore, as Cheek [24] stressed, when the research is conducted in a specific setting, among a specified group of people, as in the case of the current study, anonymity might be difficult to ensure. The researchers therefore paid special attention to protect the anonymity and confidentiality of the participants. To protect anonymity of the participants, pseudonyms were used throughout the research process and in the final report of the study. Assurances were given to participants by the researchers that any information gained during the interview would be held in the strictest confidence. In addition, the researchers guaranteed the anonymity of participants in any reports or publications generated as a result of this study.

Confidentiality between the participants and the researchers was assured by meeting the participants in a safe environment. The time of the interviews was always scheduled to suit the participants. All data were dated and labelled with pseudonyms to avoid identification of participants or in the event of loss or theft. The data were kept in a password- protected computer, and all tapes and written notes generated were placed in a locked cabinet, the key being held by the researchers.

3.5. Data collection, management and analysis

The aim of this research study was discovering a phenomenon in a social context; therefore, to gather rich data in order to generate a strong grounded theory, unstructured interviews were found as the most appropriate data collection technique, as it permits exploration of how midwifery students perceive intimate touch in clinical practice. The inclusion criteria for the participants were the following: third year midwifery student at the University of Ljubljana and Faculty of Health Sciences who finished all clinical practice. Each participant was a volunteer. McNamara [25] points out that interviews are particularly useful for getting the story behind a participant's experiences and that the interviewer can pursue in-depth information around the topic. Face- to- face interviews were conducted over the period of 2 months that consisted of nine in- depth and open-ended questions. The interviews lasted from 15 to 25 minutes and were audio taped from the beginning till the end. The tapes were labelled using the participants' pseudonyms. After the interview, researchers relistened to the recorded conversations, and the interviews were transcribed as verbatim as possible.

In grounded theory (as described by Liehr and LoBiondo – Wood) [26], data analysis proceeds through several levels and comprises several distinctive features which assist the research process. They are theoretical sensitivity, theoretical sampling and saturation, coding and categorizing the data and theoretical memos.

As Bluff [23] describes, the sample size in a grounded theory study tends to be small. According to Straus and Corbin [13], the key to grounded theory is to generate enough in-depth data that can illuminate patterns, concepts, categories, properties and dimensions of the given phenomena. Theoretical saturation occurs when no new or relevant data seem to emerge regarding a category, and, as Strauss and Corbin [13] pointed out, the category is well developed in terms of its properties and dimensions, demonstrating variation and the relationship among categories, which are well established and validated. In the current study, the saturation occurred with the sample size of nine participants. Data collection and analysis were ongoing throughout the research and involved three steps: open coding to find categories, axial coding to find links between the themes/categories and selective coding to find the core category which explained the phenomenon that was emerging from the study.

4. Findings and discussion

This chapter is providing an overview of the findings that gave rise to the theory. The properties and dimensions of the core category emerged slowly. The core category **Feeling abused and being the abuser** allowed the researchers to refine a conceptual theory to explain all the categories and their interrelationships.

The three categories relate to the core category, which is the central phenomenon and, at the same time, the main concern of third year midwifery students in Slovenia. The core category **Feeling abused and being the abuser** is broad in range and is able to integrate end explain the relationship between the key categories. Because of the unprofessional attitude towards women and students and between clinical mentors, many boundaries are being crossed, and as a consequence, the quality of being worthy of respect of all involved is being compromised.

If a woman doesn't allow for students to be present (pause), well, I think she has a reason for it and I am not going to that room! But then the clinical mentor forces you to go in saying "put your badge to

http://dx.doi.org/10.5772/60499

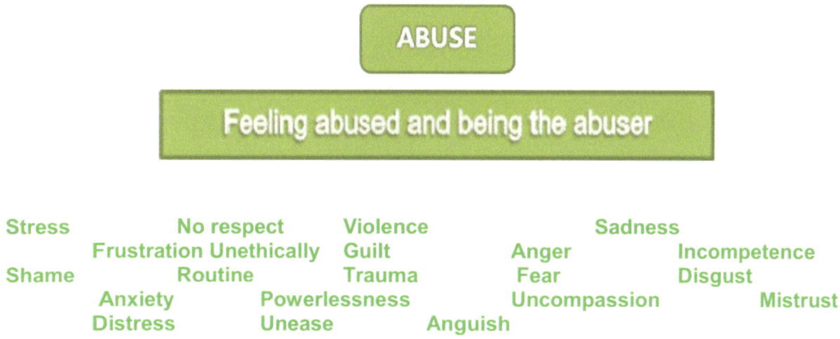

Figure 2. The core category, the three conceptual categories and their concepts

your pocket and go, the women won't even know that you are a student!" and that makes it even worse. At that point (pause) just checking the uterus (pause) it's hard... you have a feeling that you are violating her (pause) with your presence, with your hypocrisy doing something the mentor told you to do. (Lila)

Midwives are supposed to be supportive, empathic and acting as advocates for women. The environment in which they are working should be such that the midwife is, as Field [27] stresses, able to expect the support and empathy from colleagues. This is even more important when a midwife is also a mentor to midwifery students who are sent to clinical practice. The desirable mentor qualities, as pointed out by NHS [28], are – among other qualities, personal characteristics and behaviours – acting as a role model, awareness of own practice and positive attitude towards students.*It was in the first year when we had clinical practice in the delivery room, I was assigned to work with an older midwife, and she was also my clinical mentor. She told me nothing, she kept leaving me alone in the room. When I asked her something she answered in a rude manner. I was on my own, scared and I remember I was forced (by that mentor) to give an enema to a woman who didn't want it. (Zarja)*

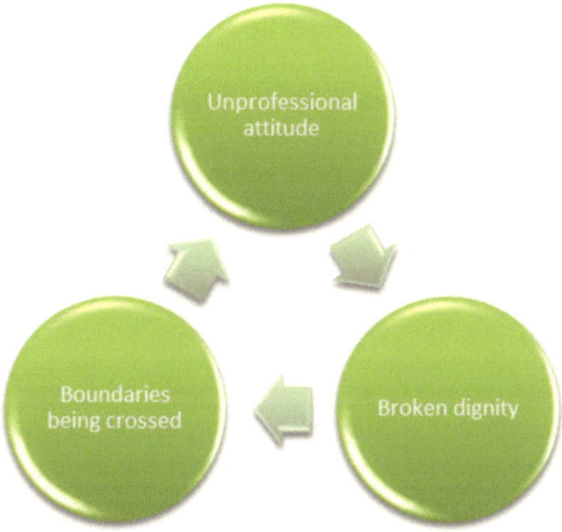

Figure 3. The circle of the key categories

The above- mentioned categories rounds around and define the core category. Unprofessional attitude, boundaries being crossed and broken dignity were found to have a central consequence, which is the statement that midwifery students at clinical practice, when they are dealing with intimacy/intimate touch, are feeling abused and, at the same time, feel that they are the abusers. The theory is true to real life, as it explains how midwifery students perceive their experience of intimacy in clinical practice and what is their most typical experience of intimate touch in clinical practice and is clearly understandable to participants, educators and health care professionals.

4.1. Unprofessional attitude

The category **Unprofessional attitude** considers the importance of informed consent, the seriousness of communication failures, the fact of lost assertiveness and the presence of fatigue and apathy.

Every medical examination might be considered as an intimate event. Assessing the location of the fundus of the uterus can be just as intimate as examining the eye. Therefore, all procedures in health care need to be based on informed consent. Intimate examination and all sources of treatments can be a source of distress and discomfort to women. It is crucial that midwives and midwifery students are well aware that a competent adult has a right to respect for his autonomy, which includes protection of his bodily integrity. The patient's right to autonomy should always be respected, and steps need to be taken to make consent truly informed [29].*No, I am not asking for real...I don't think I am asking for real...I explain what we are going to do, and how it is going to be done, sometimes even why....in matter of fact if a women doesn't answer to my explanation I take her silence as a consent... (Jona)*

Students aim to respect their patient's wishes and preferences, though when the patient's preference cannot be maintained, they provide intimate care as an essential activity of daily living [30]. However, this could be counterproductive, as the midwives' fitness to practice could be challenged when providing care without full consent [31]. A principal general practitioner wrote her personal experience of intimate examination, emphasizing how the informed consent failed to protect her. She described her experience: 'I was admitted to hospital. Preoperatively, 12-20 people in white came to examine me. I did not realize, but medical students could examine patients unsupervised, as I assumed they were doctors. They all performed chest and abdominal examinations. Three performed breast examination. All performed vaginal or rectal examinations. Three performed both, which was particularly distressing. Consent was obtained in the form of "if you don't mind, I need to,"...and I consented by my physical position and embarrassed "OK." I felt upset, vulnerable and unclean. After the first three examinations I wanted to go home, but I still consented.'

No one prepared us for this intimate touching when we are at clinical practice. I always ask a woman if I can touch her but I never wait for her permission, for her saying:" yes, you can touch me" I just do it. (Nika)

The frequent requirement of midwives to touch patients in intimate or sensitive areas often causes distress and embarrassment to patients. To protect patients from inhuman or degrading treatments, the law requires that they are only carried out where medically necessary by a suitably qualified person and if possible accompanied by a chaperone to oversee the procedure [32].

In situations where the woman-midwife partnership may not be apparent within midwifery, there can be an acknowledged power imbalance present in a professional relationship that places each woman, her infant(s) and her family in a position of potential vulnerability and of potential exposure to exploitation or abuse if that trust is not respected. The trust placed in the midwife by the woman and her family is essential to enable the midwife to provide comprehensive, effective and supportive care to the woman, her infant(s) and her family. Maintaining that level of trust is the responsibility of all midwives. This means the midwife takes responsibility for, and is accountable for, maintaining professional and personal boundaries as well as assisting colleagues and the women in their care in maintaining theirs. Health care professionals need to seek permission from patients prior to touch and conclude that 'significant component of the propriety if touch is related to patient consent'. Sadly, O'Lynn and Krautscheid [33] believe that most employers don't require nurses or midwives to obtain formal consent from patients before performing any task requiring intimate touch.

For the delivery of high- quality and safe care, it is essential to use effective communication [34, 35]; unfortunately, effective communication is all too frequently personality dependent.

I feel burdened because I know the communication and terminology is completely inappropriate: "push like you are going to poop and pee-pee, good girl)...", unpleasant (pause), inappropriate....(Dora)

Midwifery students realize that the communication between midwives and women is often inappropriate. These so- called communication failures are, as Leonard et al. [35] pointed out, an extremely common cause of inadvertent patient harm; therefore, it is critically important that health care providers create an environment in which individuals can speak up and express concerns to alert to unsafe situations. Nonverbal communication is one aspect of communication and is defined as a variety of communicative behaviours that do not carry linguistic content [36]. It can be described as a gesture, touch, posture, facial expression, eye contact, etc. [37]. A great amount of nonverbal communication can be seen in midwifery work. It is used to express and communicate thoughts, feelings and emotions and to establish and maintain a relationship.

Sometimes they (older mentors) simply come into the room give same instructions, (pause) "empty words and this is it. They don't even look into their eyes. (Nora)

Clinical mentors don't think about this (intimate touch) much. They don't respect the intimacy and privacy of a woman...and you are chough somewhere in between the mentors' demands and the women's wishes (sighs) if you want to survive you simply need to "switch" of. (Dora).

The 'switching off' is a passive behaviour, which can lead to manipulative behaviour. Students are, because of the pressure of gathering the expectant number of procedures, pushed into the situation where they manipulate with women. If the mentors are not providing safe and supportive care, neither are the students. As Fowler [38] pointed out, midwifery mentors have various opinions of professional accountability, depending on personal experience, which consequently influences student protégés accordingly.*I was missing a few vaginal check-ups... A midwife told me to go and get them....I said to the woman I was going to do a vaginal check-up... the woman replied that she had been checked-up downstairs (at triage) but I insisted as these check-ups are made also here despite being examined half an hour earlier (pause) honestly I didn't want to do it... I didn't want to... but I felt the pressure... that reaction of hers... I saw she was hardly waiting to pass, hardly waiting for me to finish and leave the room. (Nora)*

Students were unable to act assertive. They were not able to express themselves with confidence and without having to resort to passive, aggressive or manipulative behaviour, which is, as Bishop [39] states, assertiveness. Assertiveness can also be defined as a core interpersonal behaviour and a key to human relations [40]. It is a skill and capacity of interpersonal communication [41] that can be taught [27]. The problem occurs when a midwife, who is at the same time a clinical mentor, loses her assertiveness. An assertion cycle is a tool to guide and improve assertion in the interest of patient safety.

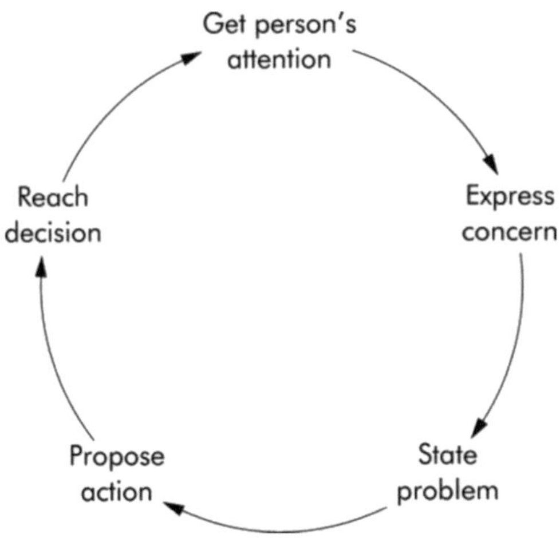

Figure 4. Assertion cycle [35]

The social influence of behaviour, which means that the behaviour of one person affects the behaviour of another person, was described by more than one participant.

If you want to survive, you have to start acting like them (mentors) (Dora).

The statement above is an apparent sign of apathy and fatigue, which is a reality in health care. Weinstein [42] points out that fatigue is not only mental or physical exhaustion and that the person might feel tired through physical and mental effort. It is undeniable that midwifery work is physically, but mostly mentally and emotionally, demanding.

It is hard. The women doesn't thrust you, the mentor doesn't, thrust you, you don't thrust yourself, because you don't,' know what you are doing.... (Lila)

The participants themselves showed indicators of fatigue and apathy as they exhibited lack of energy and intention, poor decision- making, lack of initiative and poor communication.

...at the beginning of a study you think all the time about how the person feels, what she is going through. Later on, you become like a robot.... (Lila)

A responsibility of every one who works in health care is to take over the responsibility for fatigue and to find balance between personal and professional life. Students should be protected from too much stress and offered ongoing support by their clinical mentors. It is alarming that students feel fatigue and apathy.

4.2. Boundaries being crossed

The category **Boundaries being crossed** considers the students' experiences of negative emotions and their ambivalent attitudes towards intimacy and a naked body and the vulnerability of all involved.

Boundaries bring order to humans' lives; they empower and protect an individual from the ignorance, meanness and thoughtlessness of others. There are several types of boundary violations:

- The intrusion violation
- The distance violation
- Physical boundaries
- Emotional boundaries
- Ethical boundaries
- Professional boundaries

A midwife, who is at the same time clinical mentor to midwifery students, may, among other things, violate a boundary in terms of physical contact, intimacy, disclosure, etc. Even though some boundaries are clear cut, all boundary violations are extremely complex. There are two types of professional boundary matters: boundary crossings and boundary violations. Boundary crossings are described as brief excursions across professional boundaries that may be inadvertent, thoughtless or even purposeful. Boundary violations refer to the misuse of power or the betrayal of trust, respect or intimacy between a midwife and a woman [43]. Morrall [44] points out that students are thought of as 'the bottom of the pile' and, because of their desire to become part of the team and to become accepted, can overtake their learning experience. It is a fact that within clinical environments, there is a hierarchy in the workplace, which can create an inferiority complex and fuel the adoption of bad behaviour.

Within the midwife/clinical mentor – woman – student relationship, the woman and the student are often vulnerable, because the midwife is in the position of power. When a student is observing the boundary crossing and boundary violations or he himself is being exposed to it, he is in jeopardy of developing negative emotions such as fear, guilt, shame, anger, anxiety, disgust sadness, doubt, etc.

At that point I felt like we didn't do all we were supposed to do, to protect the woman's intimacy...there is this feeling of responsibility, guilt. (Nika)

Childbirth itself is an emotional event for all involved: the woman, her partner, the midwife and, if present, the midwifery student. The emotions can be both profoundly positive and, unfortunately, also deeply traumatic.

...I told her (woman) that we are going to do vaginal examination every hour. Instantly I noted that something isn't ok....she told me that she was raped as a child by her father...I ensured her that we will do everything to protect her, that we will minimize the number of exams. I told the mentor about it....the mentor didn't give much attention to it and just continue with the routine procedures. After her doing the vaginal examination the woman didn't want the doctor to do another vaginal examination.... the doctor ignored her request and literally pushed her fingers inside her....at that point I left the room, I couldn't be there anymore, I am still having bad dreams. I heard the woman screaming: Leave me alone, I don't want this, you are hurting me and the doctor: "relax we are just trying to help you". Horrible...horrible (pause) I stud there feeling terrible wishing to disappear... (Lila).

This deeply traumatic experience of one of the participants shows the intricacy of contact while accomplishing routine clinical tasks. Midwives most often 'get through the work' by focusing on task- oriented aspects of care, and much of the learning of midwifery students still takes place 'on the job', whereby students learn to manage emotion by adopting a task-oriented approach to care [45]. Students often feel challenged and intimidated to provide intimate care in the health care setting, as they are faced with social, professional, academic and peer expectations and experience high levels of stress when providing intimate care [30].*Vaginal examination was one of the worst things for me. You are reaching so deeply in to the intimacy of a woman. I am always wondering how the husband deals with this, because I am feeling extremely unpleasant invading the privacy of his wife's vagina. (Nora)*

Senior midwives seem to retain their dominant position by means of unwritten rules, which are often idiosyncratic and most common in the accounts of student midwives, who are making the transition from being 'outsiders' in midwifery to 'insiders' and are keenly aware that senior midwives are the gatekeepers to this passage. Furthermore, students are especially vulnerable in this respect, as it is the senior midwives who assess their clinical ability [46].*Every time I feel so scared and nervous. I am hoping that everything goes well and that the woman won't comment on me and my work in front of my mentor. (Jona)*

According to Crossan and Mathew [30], students aim to achieve a balance between their own comfort and discomfort levels versus the woman's level of comfort and discomfort when providing intimate care. In the model of intimate care situations affecting comfort and discomfort in women and the care provider, both the student and the patient are likely to move in and out of their comfort end discomfort zones.*For several times I have asked myself how do they feel about me being present at this intimate event (birth)? Do they like me or do they have a bad feeling when I'm looking and touching their vaginas, breasts, perineum.... (Nika)*

The participants perceive the intimate touch as a stressful event for them and for women. They are aware of the vulnerability of all involved.

For me, the first vaginal examination was very stressful, as it was very painful for the woman. I felt as I did something bad to her. Afterwards I had to sit and drink a glass of water. (Ina)

All involved in midwifery education need to know how to manage student stress effectively. As pointed out by Pryjmachuk and Richards [47], this can be achieved by ensuring that personal teachers play a key role in supporting students, especially when students self-report high levels of stress.

4.3. Broken dignity

Broken dignity is the category that highlights the importance of understanding how invading someone's intimacy can be a human rights violation and, therefore, an exploitation or an abuse.

Dignity is a global concern in health care and fundamental for every patient. To lose dignity means that a person has been exposed in ways that affected his worth [48]. There has been a growing interest in, and concern about, dignity, or, rather, the lack of it, in care services [49]. Quality of care includes quality of caring, and this means how personal care is the compassion, dignity and respect with which patients are treated.*Today there was a woman giving birth and the door was open. Me and my colleague were passing by... they simply don't close the door and they don't' respect the intimacy. And those terrible hospital attendants... in and out of the room. (INA)*

Midwives, whose roles bring them into intimate contact with others, can easily undermine women's self-worth, usually through sheer thoughtlessness such as neglecting to close the door [48].

Mentors should be role models for their students [50] and should never put the students in the position where they are forced to invade another person's intimacy.

It depends on the department... and experience of the supervisor... the longer her career lasts, the less sensitive she becomes for woman's dignity and her intimacy. (LILA)

Invading intimacy is also an area of concern for midwifery students. They understand that, for many women, vaginal examinations bring up issues of sexual intimacy, invasion of privacy and vulnerability [51].*I don't want to do serial vaginal examinations as well...I feel how vulnerable are women at that point. (Petja)*

There is also a concern of violation of human rights when invading into another person's intimacy, as human rights and human dignity are intimately linked [52]. As Sulmasy [52] points out, all human rights depend upon the concept of human dignity. The right not to be experimented upon without consent is an absolute human right in health care.

The most terrible for me is giving enema or doing vaginal check-up, shavings... as I know they feel terribly as they are already explaining in advance »I am shaved« or »I'm not shaved«... (SARA)

It is the responsibility of a clinical mentor to protect the dignity of a woman and of a student. All midwives should act upon a code of ethics. The Slovenian Midwifery Code of Ethics (Kodeks etike za babice) [53] acknowledges women as persons with human rights, seeks justice for all people and equity in access to health care, and is based on mutual relationships of respect and trust and the dignity of all members of society.

5. Conclusion and recommendations

The findings of this study are somewhat disturbing, because it is quite clear that midwifery students are not appropriately prepared for the intensity of intimacy and emotions related to their work at clinical practice. The students are classified as young adult s, but they might still be in a process of looking for their identity and, consequently, still building their personality. It is well known that young persons' sexuality is about growing awareness, experience and expression of eroticism, sexual pleasure, intimacy, sexual orientation and gender identity. It is less known that it is also about the social rules, economic structures, political battles and religious ideologies that surround physical expressions of intimacy and the relationships within which such intimacy takes place [54].

In a way, this study opened Pandora's box. But, even though, by definition, this means to get into a situation over which one has very little control or to create an uncontrollable situation that will cause great grief, the researchers believe it was a box that needed and was meant to be opened. The midwifery students in clinical settings and the women who are seeking help, advice or care from health care professionals need to be protected from abuse of all kinds.

All students, while on practice placements, should be supported and assessed by a registered practitioner, who has undertaken an approved mentor preparation programme, with mentors expected to support, facilitate learning and assess the clinical competence of pre-registration students within the practice setting [55].

It is apparent that very few midwifery textbooks cover the topic of intimate touch and very few midwifery curricula focus on the complexity of intimate touch; therefore, midwifery students gain their skills by trial and error in clinical practice, which is far from appropriate. The researchers noted that students give great thought to intimacy issues while on their clinical practice and that they fear that their touch will be misinterpreted, and from the literature review, it is clear that many women have mixed feelings about intimate touch provided by students. Therefore, midwifery students should have the possibility to reflect on how they understand, perceive and approach intimate touch. Midwifery education should be based on the development of evidence- based strategies for intimate touch, and midwifery educators should consider discussing with students the anxiety and uncertainty that they feel when providing intimate touch.

The researchers believe that, regarding this study, it is not enough to write only a conclusion and recommendations, but it is necessary to act proactive. Therefore, one of the researchers, who also has a degree in marriage and family therapy, will use her knowledge of counselling and start an assertiveness training programme, which focuses on how to react to difficult interactions in daily life for midwifery students in order to help the individual change how they view themselves, improve their assertiveness, properly express their individual moods and thoughts and further establish self-confidence. Lin et al. [56] found out that the assertiveness training programme significantly increased the assertiveness and self-esteem of students, especially among individuals with low assertiveness and self-esteem.

The development of a theoretical framework and evidence - based strategies regarding intimate examination would be of benefit to the clinical practice, supervision and education of midwifery students. It would provide students with the best possible educational experience and an optimal midwifery care to women. The conflict between educational needs and ethical requirements is especially acute in the teaching of intimate examinations. The teaching of intimate examinations poses ethical problems, not only for the student but also for educators, because students must learn, but patients must be protected [57].

The methodology used in this study provided a unique insight into the perception of Slovenian midwifery students on intimate touch in clinical practice. The findings of our study cannot be generalized but can help in building up the awareness of the importance of the issues of sexuality and intimacy in midwifery. Clearly, there are implications for further research on the topic of intimate touch, which should include women's perspective as well as the perspectives of mentors and faculty educators.

Author details

Tita Stanek Zidarič* and Metka Skubic

*Address all correspondence to: tita.zidaric@zf.uni-lj.si

University of Ljubljana, Faculty of Health Sciences, Midwifery Department, Slovenia

References

[1] Reis HT, Shaver P. Intimacy as interpersonal process. In: Duck S (ed.) Handbook of personal relationships: Theory, relationships, and intervention. Chichester: Wiley; 1988. p367-389.

[2] Hunter B. Emotion work in midwifery: a review of current knowledge. Journal of Advanced Nursing 2001; 34(4): 436-444.

[3] Laurenceau JP, Rivera LM., Schaffer AR, Pietromonaco PR. Intimacy as an Interpersonal Process: Current Status and Future Directions. In: Mashek DJ, Aron A (eds.) Handbook on Closeness and Intimacy. New Jersey: Lawrence Erlbaum Associates; 2004. p61-80.

[4] Harding T, et.al. Sexualizing men's touch: male nurses and the use of intimate touch in clinical practice. Res Theory Nurs Pract. 2008; 22(2): 88-102.

[5] O'Lynn C, Krautscheid L. How Should I Touch You? A Qualitative Study of Attitudes on intimate Touch in Nursing Care. AJN 2011; 111 (3).

[6] Brunstad A, Hjälmhult E. Midwifery students learning experiences in labor wards: A grounded theory. Nurse Education Today 2014 – article in press.

[7] Gould D. Quality care is more than a set of processes. British journal of midwifery 2009; 17(4): 210.

[8] Elcigil A, Sari HY. Students' opinions about and expectations of effective nursing clinical mentors. Journal of Nursing Education 2008; 47(3):118-123.

[9] Nettleton P, Bray L. Current mentorship schemes might be doing our students a disservice. Nurse Education in Practice 2008; 8: 205-212.

[10] Crossan M, Mathew TK. Exploring sensitive boundaries in nursing education: Attitudes of undergraduate student nurses providing intimate care to patients. Nurse Education in Practice 2013; 13: 317- 322.

[11] Walker SH, Davis G. Knowledge and reported confidence of final year midwifery students regarding giving advice on contraception and sexual health. Midwifery 2014; 30: 169 -176.

[12] Rees C. Introduction to Research for Midwives. (2nd ed.) Edinburgh: Books for Midwives; 2003.

[13] Strauss A, Corbin J. Basics of qualitative research: Grounded theory procedures and techniques. Newbury Park: Sage Publications; 1990.

[14] Hall HG, McKenna LG., Griffiths DL. Applaying grounded theory to midwifery research problems. International Journal of Childbirth 2012; 2 (2):136 -141.

[15] Glaser B G, Strauss AL. The discovery of grounded theory: strategies for qualitative research. New Brunswick: Aldine Transaction; 1999.

[16] Morse JM. "Situating grounded theory within qualitative inquiry" In: Schreibe RS, Stern PN. (eds.) Using Grounded Theory in Nursing. New York: Springer Publishing; 2001. p1-15.

[17] Creswell JW. Research Design: Qualitative, Quantitative, and Mixed Approaches.(4th ed.) London: SAGE Publications; 2012.

[18] Douglas D. Grounded theories of management: a methodological review. Management Research News 2003; 26 (5): 45-52.

[19] Silverman D. Doing Qualitative Research. (4th ed.) London: Sage Publications; 2010.

[20] Cahana A, Hurst SA. Voluntary informed consent in research and clinical care: an update. Pain Pract. 2008; 8(6): 446-51.

[21] Holloway I. Basic Concepts for Qualitative Research. Oxford: Blackwell science; 2004.

[22] Holloway I. Wheeler S. Qualitative Research in Nursing. Oxford: Blackwell Science; 2002.

[23] Bluff R. Grounded theory. In: Cluett ER, Bluff R. (eds.) Principles and Practice of Research in Midwifery, Edinburgh: Bailliere Tindall; 2004. p.113 -129.

[24] Cheek J. The practice and politics on funded qualitative research. In: Denzin NK, Lincoln YS (eds.) The Sage Handbook of Qualitative Research. (3rd ed.) Thousand Oaks: Sage Publications; 2005. p. 387-410.

[25] McNamara C. Field Guide to Consulting and Organizational Development: A Collaborative and Systems Approach to Performance, Change and Learning. Minnesota: Authenticity Consulting; 2006.

[26] Liehr PR, LoBiondo – Wood G. Qualitative approaches to research. In: LoBiondo – Wood G, Haber J. (eds.) Nursing Research: Methods and Critical Appraisalfor Evidence – Based Practice. (5th ed.) St. Louis: Mosby Elsevier; 2006. pp. 148- 175.

[27] Field H. Bullying and assertiveness. In: Chapman V. Charles C. (ed.) The Midwife's Labour and Birth Handbook. Oxford: Wiley-Blackwell; 2009. p299 -303.

[28] NHS Education for Scotland. National Approach to Mentor Preparation for Nurses and Midwives: Core Curriculum Framework (2nd ed.). Edinburgh: NHS Education for Scotland; 2013. http://www.nes.scot.nhs.uk/education-and-training/by-discipline/nursing-and-midwifery/practice-education/national-approach-to-mentor-preparation-2nd-edition-2013.aspx (accessed 20 February 2015).

[29] Selinger CP. The right to consent: is it absolute? British Journal of Medical Practitioners 2009; 2(2): 50 -54.

[30] Crossan M, Mathew TK. Exploring sensitive boundaries in nursing education: Attitudes of undergraduate student nurses providing intimate care to patients. Nurse Education in Practice 2013; 13: 317- 322.

[31] Nursing and Midwifery Council. Chaperoning. Retrieved 3rd September 2012. http://www.nmc-uk.org/Nurses-and-midwives/Regulation-in-practice/Regulation-in-Practice Topics/Chaperoning-/ (accessed 20th October, 2014).

[32] Griffith R. Legal requirements for conducting intimate examinations and treatments. British Journal of Midwifery 2007;15 (11): 722 -723.

[33] O'Lynn C, Krautscheid L. Original research: 'how should I touch you?': a qualitative study of attitudes on intimate touch in nursing care. Am J Nurs 2011; 111(3): 24-31.

[34] Van Servellen GM. Communication Skills for the Health Care Professional: Concepts, Practice and Evidence (2nd ed). Sudbury: Jones and Bartlett Publishing;2009.

[35] Leonard M, Graham S., Bonacum D. The human factor: the critical importance of effective teamwork and communication in providing safe care. Qual Saf Health Care 2004;13: 85-90.

[36] Knapp, ML, Hall JA. Nonverbal Communication in Human Interaction (5th ed.). Wadsworth: Thomas Learning; 2007.

[37] Finset A, Del Piccolo L. Nonverbal Communication in Clinical Contexts. Communication in Cognitive Behavioral Therapy: Springer; 2011:107-128.

[38] Fowler D. Student midwives and accountability: are mentors good role models? British Journal of Midwifery 2013; 16 (2): 100-104.

[39] Bishop S. Develop Your Assertiveness (3rd ed.). London: Kogan Page; 2013.

[40] Lin YR, Shiah IS, Chang YC, Lai TY, Wang KY, Chou KR. Evaluation of an assertiveness training program on nursing and medical students' assertiveness, self-esteem, and interpersonal communication satisfaction. Nurse Education Today 2004; 24(8): 656-665.

[41] Kim Y. The effects of assertiveness training on enhancing the social skills of adolescents with visual impairments. Journal of Visual Impairment & Blindness 2003;97(5): 285-297

[42] Weinstein SM. Fatigue. In: Weinstein SM. (ed.) B Is For Balance : 12 Steps towards a More Balanced Life At Home and At Work (2nd ed.). Indianapolis: Sigma Theta Tau International; 2014. p143-170.

[43] The Nursing and Midwifery Board of Australia (National Board). A midwife's guide to professional boundaries was first published in February 2010. Melbourne: Nursing and Midwifery Board of Australia; 2010.

[44] Morrall PA. Quality assurance in nurse education. The social context of learning. Nurse Education Today 2005; 25: 620-24.

[45] Hunter B. Emotion work in midwifery: a review of current knowledge. Journal of Advanced Nursing 2001; 34(4), 436-444.

[46] Hunter B. Emotion work and boundary maintenance in hospital-based midwifery. Midwifery 2005; 21: 253-266.

[47] Pryjmachuk S., Richards DA. Predicting stress in pre-registration midwifery students attending a university in Northern England. Midwifery 2008; 24 (1): 108-122.

[48] Matiti MR. The importance of dignity in healthcare. In: Matiti MR, Baillie L. (eds.) Dignity in Healthcare: A Practical Approach for Nurses and Midwives. London: Radclife Publishing; 2011. p3-8.

[49] Hewison A. Dignity as a policy issue in healthcare. In: Matiti MR, Baillie L (eds.) Dignity in Healthcare: A Practical Approach for Nurses and Midwives. London: Radcliffe Publishing; 2011. p37-51.

[50] Eller L, Lev E, Feurer A. Key components of an effective mentoring relationship: A qualitative study. Nurse education Today 2014; 34: 815-820.

[51] Warren C. Why should I do vaginal examinations? Practising Midwife 1999; 2: 12-13.

[52] Sulmasy DP. Dignity, Rights, Health Care, and Human Flourishing. In: Weisstub DN, Díaz Pintos G. (eds.) Autonomy and Human Rights in Health Care: An International Perspective. Dordrecht: Springer; 2008. P25- 36.

[53] Kodeks etike za babice. Ljubljana: Sekcija medicinskih sester - babic Slovenije; 2011.

[54] Coleman J., Roker D. Adolescent Sexuality and Adult Professional Behaviour: Future Directions for Policy and Practice. In: Coleman J., Roker D. (eds.) Teenage Sexuality: Health, Risk and Education. New York: Routledge; 2008. P189 -202.

[55] Nursing and Midwifery Council. Standards to Support Learning and Assessment in Practice (2nd ed.) NMC: London; 2008.

[56] Lin YR., Shiah IS., ChangYC., Lai TY., Wang KY., Chou KR. Evaluation of an assertiveness training program on nursing and medical students' assertiveness, self-esteem, and interpersonal communication satisfaction. Nurse Education Today 2004; 24(8): 656-665.

[57] Coldicott Y., Pope C., Roberts C. The ethics of intimate examinations – teaching tomorrow's doctors. BJM 2003: 326; 97-101.

Chapter 5

Sexual Activity during Pregnancy in Childbirth and after Childbirth

Teja Škodič Zakšek

Additional information is available at the end of the chapter

http://dx.doi.org/10.5772/59496

1. Introduction

According to the World Health Organization (WHO) [1] sexual health is a complex biological and sociological concept that requires a positive and responsible approach to sexuality and sexual relationships. It cannot be merely defined as the absence of sexual dysfunction. Sexual health can be greatly altered during pregnancy, birth and the postpartum period.

This chapter discusses selected important issues in sexual health during pregnancy, birth and the postpartum period. Pregnancy is a period where many physical and psychological changes occur. Such changes influence couples' lives in many ways, and their sexual life changes. Healthy sexuality during pregnancy appears to be a key stage in the evolution of a couple towards becoming parents. Sexual activity is reported to decrease throughout pregnancy, and the prevalence of reduced sexual interest and enjoyment in this period is over 60% [2]. Decreased sexual activity may be attributable to nausea, fear of miscarriage, fear of harming the foetus, lack of interest, discomfort, physical awkwardness, and fear of membrane rupture, fear of infection or fatigue or others [3].

Sexual activity is known to have an effect on the spontaneous onset of labour. This effect is thought to be due to the presence of prostaglandin E in human semen, which matures the cervix and initiates uterine contractions; the female orgasm with the liberation of oxytocin, which is responsible for uterine contractions; and breast stimulation, which initiates the oxytocin release reflex [3]. Although the effect of sexual activity in reducing the risk of prolonged pregnancies has been well documented, less is known concerning its potential consequences on the prognosis of labour [3]. Many pregnant women (and some physicians) believe that sexual intercourse at term will have an impact on the onset of labour. However, recent studies show that sexual intercourse at term is not associated with ripening of the cervix and does not hasten labour [4].

Postpartum sexual function is influenced by the many significant changes in anatomy, hormonal milieu, family structure, and partner relationships that accompany childbirth [5], yet women's experiences of postpartum sexuality have rarely been explored beyond physical dimensions and focus mostly on issues related to pregnancy, vaginal trauma and breastfeeding [6].

Despite the lack of large well designed studies on the discussed topic, the evidence available so far shows that pregnancy, childbirth and the postpartum period determine a relevant, even if reversible, negative effect on sexuality. Sexual health during pregnancy, birth and the postpartum period is increasingly being recognized as an important component of women's lives and an important area of maternity service provision, and therefore deserves our greater attention.

2. Sexual activity during pregnancy

Pregnancy is a period where many physical and psychological changes occur. Such changes influence couples' lives in many ways. Hormonal, physical and social changes commonly impact on women's physical wellbeing, mood, relationships and sexuality.

Sexual activity is reported to decrease throughout pregnancy, and the prevalence of reduced sexual interest and enjoyment in this period could be over 50% [2, 3]. Changes in the sexual life of a pregnant couple usually come gradually. Meta-analysis from von Sydow [7] and a study from Pauleta et al. [8] both demonstrated that sexuality does not significantly change in the first trimester and is slightly altered in the second trimester of pregnancy; however, the third trimester of pregnancy showed more than a 50% decrease in sexual activity [8] compared with prepregnancy states.

Decreasing sexual activity during pregnancy may be attributable to nausea, fear of miscarriage, fear of harming the foetus, lack of interest, discomfort, physical awkwardness, and fear of membrane rupture, fear of infection or fatigue or other factors which will be presented in the next subchapters.

What researchers have noticed is that sexual life during pregnancy is rarely discussed between pregnant couples and their midwives or doctors, although most women feel it should be discussed and wish to receive more information about it [9].

2.1. Social, cultural factors and norms, fears and myths

Social and cultural factors and related myths can influence the sexual life of a pregnant couple. Demographic factors such as education level, full time employment, and duration of marriage and ethnic group have been reported to influence sexual function during pregnancy [9, 10, 11]. Tosun Güleroğlu and Gördeles Beşer [10] wanted to evaluate sexual functions of pregnant women and to determine the factors that negatively affect their sexual health, determining that the sexual lives of the pregnant women were negatively affected by factors such as old age, low educational status, and arranged marriages lasting for more than ten years. They gathered data using a personal information form and the Female Sexual Function Index (FSFI)[1] from

http://dx.doi.org/10.5772/59496

over 300 participants, and also found out that 88.9% of their participants had sexual desire disorders, 86.9% had sexual arousal disorder, 42.8% had lubrication disorders, 69.6% had orgasm disorders, and 48% had sexual satisfaction disorders. Chang et al. [11] wanted to examine overall sexual function in Taiwanese women during the three trimesters of pregnancy and discovered that full time work has a significant negative effect on overall sexual function and on engagement in sexual activity during the second trimester of pregnancy.

There are numerous different sexual practices during pregnancy based on cultural factors, myths and norms, usually depending on where the couple comes from. A study by Naim and Bhutto [12] in Pakistani women revealed a decline in sexual function during pregnancy due to the belief that sexual intercourse might harm the baby, induce preterm labour and even cause abortion. Adinma [13] investigated the sexual behaviour and beliefs of 440 pregnant women from southeastern Nigeria. The mean frequency of sexual intercourse during pregnancy [1.5 times per week) was less than that before pregnancy [2.3 times per week). The husband was the main initiator of sexual activity [41.6%), while the wife was only rarely [2.7%). A total of 44.3% of the respondents believed that sexual intercourse during pregnancy widens the vagina and facilitates labour; 30.2% believed that it caused abortion in early pregnancy while 21.1% had no knowledge of any repercussions of sexual intercourse in pregnancy. In contrast to the previous mentioned study, 34.8% of women in Nigeria believed that sexual intercourse during pregnancy improves foetal wellbeing. A study among Iranian women [14] revealed their fear about sexual activity during pregnancy because of the possibility of causing rupture of the hymen of the female foetus or possible foetal blindness. They also believed sexual intercourse might be an act of adultery while carrying a female foetus. A study conducted later in the Iranian population [15] revealed that the prevalence of sexual dysfunction is high during pregnancy and reaches higher levels in the third trimester. The authors concluded that pregnant women and their partners in Iran need counselling about physical and psychological changes in pregnancy. However, teaching about harming the foetus through sexual intercourse during pregnancy is not uncommon. In China, for example, a prospective cross-sectional study [16] revealed that Chinese pregnant women had less sexual activity and desire during pregnancy. A total of 80% of 298 participants and their partners worried about the adverse effects of sexual activity on the foetus. Similarly in Taiwan a study performed by Liu, Hsu and Chen [17] explored changes in sexual experiences in pregnancy in order to identify the decrease of coital frequency in Taiwan. The majority of their subjects stopped engaging in sexual activity during pregnancy, one reason for which being the fear of harming the foetus.

Contrasting results and perceptions about having sex in pregnancy come, for example, from Poland. According to the study by Malewitz [18], sexuality in pregnancy to Polish couples means quite a stimulus to search for new ways of pleasing each other in love play. Their research makes it evident that experiencing sexual satisfaction by pregnant women improves their self-esteem, facilitates mutual relationship between partners and tightens the marital bond [18].

---

1 FSFI is a multidimensional instrument developed by Rosen et al. in the United States in 2000 in order to assess female sexual functions (6).

Regardless of the social or cultural background of a pregnant couple, their positive or their negative perceptions about sexuality in pregnancy have an influence on their sexual behaviour in this fragile time of their life.

2.2. Biomedical, psychological and relationship factors

Sexuality and problems during the transition to parenthood are influenced by a complex interplay of biomedical, psychological and relationship factors, claims von Sydow [7]. In pregnancy, female hormonal function as well as physical and psychological changes may provoke and promote decline in sexual activities.

Hormonal changes (increased oestrogen, progesterone, and prolactin) cause nausea and breast tenderness, which together with fatigue, weakness, exhaustion and anxiety can reduce sexual desire and arousal or in other ways determine the difficulty of sexual life [19]. Relaxin, for example, causes epithelia cells in the vagina to enlarge and vaginal circumference lumen to increase, and this subsequently might cause a decrease in vaginal sensitivity [20]. Recent studies also suggest that hormones cause symptoms of diminished clitoral sensation, orgasmic disorders that may last up to six months postpartum and lack of libido [21]. Some authors [22-24] correlate diminished sexual desire with sex hormone alterations, but there are no valid studies so far to prove their major impact on women's sexuality during pregnancy [21]. To be exact, in pregnancy serum androgen levels have the highest levels in the beginning of pregnancy and then they fall in the third trimester, which should theoretically lead to a decrease in sexual desire. However, this was explored by Erol et al. [25] in a cross-sectional study where no significant correlation was found. Thorne and Stuckey [26] think that if lower sexual desire towards the end of pregnancy is hormone-related, the most likely explanation is that high progestin, as seen in the experimental evidence with exogenous hormones, negatively influences sexual behaviour, rather than decreased androgen levels. Although men may not experience the hormonal changes that occur within their partners' bodies, they often have emotional and visceral reactions to the pregnancy [27].

Morning sickness and fatigue are one of the most common problems and reasons for loss of sexual desire during pregnancy. Even though weight gain is one of the normal processes in pregnancy, it has been suggested that worry about gaining fat and physical appearance is still a prominent preoccupation during pregnancy [19]. Kitzinger [28] is convinced that the nausea and vomiting many women experience during the first trimester may diminish their feelings of eroticism, and fatigue may lead to insufficient energy to participate or enjoy in sexual intercourse. There are also other physical changes, and we can only speculate as to the extent to which they influence or alter couples' sexuality. In the first trimester breasts may become quite tender and enlarged. Kitzinger [28] notes that while a male partner may find larger breasts exciting, the female partner may find any breast or nipple stimulation to be painful rather than erotic. Some investigators notice in their research an increase in frequency and responsiveness during the second trimester of pregnancy, possibly related to pelvis congestion at that time [29]. This pelvic congestion may lead to a marked increase in the intensity of a woman's orgasm. Many women who never have experienced orgasm during intercourse have

http://dx.doi.org/10.5772/59496

their first orgasms during this time; women who previously have been orgasmic may have the experience of multiple orgasms [30].

Sexual pain disorders, including vaginismus and dyspareunia, are quite prevalent in pregnancy. Results suggest that about half of women may develop genito-pelvic pain during pregnancy, which will persist for about a third, and a subset will develop this pain after childbirth [31].

Studies have shown that pregnancy involves anatomic changes to the lower genitourinary tract and pelvic floor that may result in urinary incontinence [32]. In a retrospective study of women in the general population, urinary incontinence had negative effects on sexual function, but no significant correlation between urinary symptoms and sexual function in pregnancy has so far been found [27]. However, by the third trimester physical changes of pregnancy also become obvious on the outside, and women might feel less attractive due to their increased size. Lewis [27] noticed that some couples feel as if a third person is in bed during lovemaking, which can be distracting. Foetal movements, and Braxton-Hicks contractions may serve to diminish feelings of intimacy, and the woman's increasingly large abdomen may make usual sexual practices uncomfortable or difficult [27].

Johnsson [21] says that sexual difficulties during pregnancy might be psychological in origin, occurring as an emotional response to the changed state of the woman. Naki Radoš et al. [33] examined the role of maternal body image and body image self-consciousness in sexual satisfaction and intercourse frequency during pregnancy when controlling for satisfaction with the partnership. The findings suggested that satisfaction with body image and body image self-consciousness were related to sexual satisfaction. Nevertheless, other aspects of partnership, such as communication, appeared to be much more important predictors of sexual satisfaction than body image variables [33]. There are also many other psychogenic factors that might affect women's sexual desire; besides the already mentioned fear about harming the foetus, anxiety of delivery or capability of being a good mother could also cause distress [25].

There is limited research about the psychological benefits of sexuality in pregnancy, but at least meta-analysis from von Sydow [7] has found that sexual enjoyment during pregnancy is associated with higher relationship stability, tenderness and communication at four months and three years postpartum.

2.3. Those who are at risk

There is limited evidence in advising pregnant women at risk on sexual activity. Most common risks to sexual intercourse during pregnancy are listed in Table 1.

Johnsson [21] talks about absolute and relative contraindications to sexual intercourse during pregnancy. According to her, absolute contraindications include unexplained vaginal bleeding, placenta praevia, premature dilatation of cervix and premature rupture of membranes, and relative contraindications include a history of premature delivery and multiple gestation. These indications have not been validated with the study. The author of this chapter, however, thinks it is better to talk about risk instead of contraindications. In the case of placenta praevia, for example, it has been advised not to do an examination of the cervix [34], and it has also been theorized that penile contact during intercourse could result in a similar risk of haemorrhage [35]. A study by Timor-Tritch and Yunis [36] evaluated the safety of transvaginal ultrasonography in the diagnosis of placenta praevia, by determining whether the angle between the cervix and the vaginal probe is sufficient for alignment of the probe with the cervix. In 18 cases of placenta praevia, their findings showed that the angle between the cervix and vaginal probe is sufficient to prevent the probe from inadvertently slipping into the cervix. Although the study used a small number of participants, researchers claim that their study supports the safety of transvaginal sonography in diagnosing and monitoring patients with known placenta praevia. There are no studies of alignment of penile contact with the cervix during intercourse, so we cannot, based on the Timor-Tritch and Yunis [36] study, definitely claim that some women with placenta praevia might have or not have sexual intercourse during pregnancy. Although doctors think it is the best way for women to advice to abstain from sexual intercourse [35] we should consider every case separately and evaluate how much are they at risk rather than say that sexual intercourse is contraindicated for every women with placenta praevia.

Serious risks:
• unexplained vaginal bleeding.
• placenta praevia.
• premature dilatation of cervix.
• premature rupture of membranes.
Increased risks:
• history of premature delivery.
• multiple gestation.
• repetitive bacterial vaginosis.

Table 1. Most common risks to sexual intercourse during pregnancy

There is a common misconception that pregnant woman are not at risk for developing pelvic inflammatory disease (PID) due to a mucus plug in their cervix and obliteration in the uterine cavity due to decidua capsularis and parietalis. Theoretically they are at increased risk of getting the infection [35], but when they get ill they are at greater risk due to a possible delay in treatment, which could be a hazard to pregnant women or their unborn children. There are several case reports and studies that prove that PID and pregnancy can coexist [37-40], and that treatment is much more complicated. In addition, there are also studies that have found a link between bacterial vaginosis and cervicitis, endometriosis and salpingitis [41]. Special attention should be paid when advising about sexuality to pregnant women with repetitive bacterial vaginosis, and women with no symptoms or evidence of lower genital tract infection should be reassured that sexual activity in pregnancy does not increase the risk of preterm delivery.

Although some people consider twin or higher multiple gestation pregnancies at serious risk of preterm labour as a result of sexual activity, none of the studies confirmed that. Neilson and

Mutanbira [42] studied the effect of coitus on the precipitation of preterm labour in 126 women with twin pregnancies. The data indicate that coitus is not an important precipitant of preterm labour and that coitus need not be discouraged in women with twin pregnancies. Simlar Stammler-Safar et al. [43] wanted to evaluate changes in sexual activity in women with twin pregnancies and whether a higher frequency of sexual intercourse was associated with an increased risk of pregnancy complications. Their results demonstrate a decrease in the frequency of sexual intercourse, and they found no association between sexual activity and preterm delivery.

Substantial evidence about the safety of having sexual intercourse during pregnancy in those women who are at greater risk is missing. A woman's risk of an adverse pregnancy outcome as a result of sexual intercourse should be considered separately for each individual.

2.4. Counselling

Healthy sexuality appears to be a key stage in the transition of a couple to a family [21, 44]. Problems in sexual functioning during this stage may be amplified during this period of profound physical, emotional and psychological changes [21]. Polomeno [45] discovered that the way in which a couple deals with this sensitive period could also impact on the labour and birth. However, this area needs further investigation.

A pregnant woman may come for the first time to the antenatal clinic anytime between the first and last trimester, and she may or may not return to the clinic before birth. It is imperative, therefore, to make the most of her first visit [46]. Sometimes couples are not aware of alterations in sexual functioning in pregnancy and might be frightened or having a hard time adapting to changes. Many studies exploring sexual functions of pregnant women [9-18] identified that couples do not receive adequate (if any) information about changes in their sexual functioning. Women or couples are also not always comfortable in raising sexual concerns [21]. Therefore, it is extremely important for a healthcare provider to demonstrate good counselling skills, and specific behaviours that improve communication and/or make the client feel comfortable include [46]:

- Introducing oneself before proceeding with the interviews.
- Asking permission to talk about personal or sensitive issues.
- Asking open-ended questions using simple words.
- Encouraging clients to ask questions.
- Treating clients with respect.
- Seeing clients in private.
- Assuring the client's confidentiality.

Discussing sexuality in pregnancy with the healthcare provider is well within the scope of a routine consultation. If healthcare providers are comfortable discussing sexuality and intimacy they might also help the client to feel safe to disclose other relationship issues [47]. However, patients may have difficulty talking to healthcare providers about sexuality and sexual health in pregnancy. Most people are not used to discussing sexual matters openly.

When a woman comes to her first antenatal check-up, at history-taking there are, according to Johnsson [21], several points to consider beside regular pregnancy-related issues: assessment of the relationships (sexual and otherwise), patient support network, whether the pregnancy was planned, previous outcomes of pregnancies, previous deliveries, current health, contraception (past and future), etc. Taking a patient's sexual history can facilitate a discussion on sexuality and sexual health and need not take an inordinate amount of time. Kinsberg [48] proposes the following scheme to initiate discussion of sexual issues:

- Are you or your partner having any sexual difficulties at this time?
- Are you satisfied with your current sexual relationship?
- Do you have any sexual concerns you would like to discuss?

If a patient's answers suggest that she wants to discuss sexual issues, the following questions might be productive:

- Tell me about your sexual history— first sexual experiences, masturbation, how many partners you've had, any sexually transmitted infections or sexual problems you've had, and any past sexual abuse or trauma.
- How often do you engage in sexual activity?
- What kinds of sexual activities do you engage in?
- Do you have difficulty with desire, arousal, or orgasm?

The answers to this question should give us an orientation to incorporate targeted counselling on expected changes in sexual health related to pregnancy. To facilitate effective communication with patients on sexuality and sexual health, providers should [46]:

- Promote sexual health in clinical practice environments.
- Provide patients with current information regarding sexual health.
- Acknowledge their patients' feelings, attitudes, and norms that may be obstacles to individual sexual health and use this information to help patients establish realistic goals.
- Assist patients with the development of skills they may need to achieve personal goals for sexual health (e.g., communication, negotiation, and planning strategies).
- Participate in continuing education activities focused on sexual health.
- Be aware and respectful of their patients' sexual values and lifestyles.
- Understand how values of the healthcare provider or the clinical setting may influence practices and take care to provide unbiased and comprehensive care.

Johnsson [21] is convinced that healthcare providers should reinforce the normal reduction in the frequency of sexual intercourse as well as libido, sexual desire and orgasm that commonly occur particularly until the end of the pregnancy; however, what is normal to one couple might not be normal for the other, so each case should be considered separately. It is also essential that couples know that having sexual intercourse during pregnancy is usually safe and is not harming their unborn child. Healthcare providers should also discuss other options for the expression of intimacy with couples, such as different forms of non-coital contact that could also be pleasant and satisfying for both partners.

During the following visits the healthcare provider should ask for any new things that might emerge and give advice on problems that might arise. There is a strong evidence-based argument in favour of discussing sex and relationships at every opportunity, and maternity care providers must have access to resources to provide sexual education and support, within ethical boundaries [48].

Key points:

- Sex is generally considered safe in pregnancy.
- During the last weeks of pregnancy female sexuality is universally low or non-existent [7].
- There is limited evidence of advising pregnant women at risk on sexual activity.
- In every other phase of the transition to parenthood female sexuality is very variable depending on perspective mother physical and mental health, her sexual or nonsexual history, relationship of the couple and her life circumstances [7].
- Healthy women and their partners can stay sexually active during the entire pregnancy; however, sexual activity needs to be discouraged if certain problems occur [7].
- Discussion of sexuality in pregnancy with a healthcare provider is essential for every pregnant couple and should be part of routine practice for those who are providing maternity care.

3. Sexual intercourse and/at the onset of labour, review of evidence

Many women believe that sexual intercourse at term will hasten the onset of labour. Shaffir [5] reports a study where over 73% of pregnant women knew about this concept and 46.1% believed it to be true. It is very common also for midwives and doctors to suggest sexual intercourse or love making as a means to ripen the cervix and induce labour. Even Varney's Midwifery [49], a professional midwifery text, and May Gaskin's books [50-52] as lay midwifery reading include sexual intercourse as a method for the onset of labour. But Myles textbook for midwives [53] as another important professional midwifery book says: '... insufficient data are available...' (p. 540].

It has been speculated that nipple stimulation, clitoral stimulation and uterine activity provoked by orgasm may aid initiation and augmentation in labour. The production of oxytocin and prostaglandins as a result of both is thought to provide that physiological basis [53]. Toth et al. [54], in their study, measured cervical mucus concentrations of prostaglandins E (PGE) and F (PGF) in 30 pregnant women during their entire pregnancy. During the first and second trimester, the concentrations of PGE and PGF were similar, but during the third trimester PGF levels were ten to 20 times higher. Two to four hours after intercourse, prostaglandin concentrations in the cervical mucus were found to be about ten to 50 times higher than normal. Researchers thought that the prostaglandins in cervical mucus might participate in the gradual changes in the extracellular matrix of the cervix that result in the extensive remodelling of the cervix during pregnancy [54]. F and E series prostaglandins play an important role in ripening the cervix and contribute to the contractibility of the uterus, are produced by the cervix, are known to be produced by the foetal membranes and the decidua, and are detectable in liquor in increasing quantities before term [53]. F and E series prostaglandins result in uterine contractions, E series prostaglandins are relatively more uteroselective and are clearly superior to F series prostaglandins in producing cervical ripening [55]. Increased prostaglandin concentrations in the Toth et al. [54] study could be due to the presence of semen, which contains prostaglandin. In fact, the richest source of prostaglandins in humans are indeed seminal vesicles [56]. Therefore, there is a biological plausibility regarding the effect of sexual intercourse on the onset of labour from this point of view. However, when Shaffir [5] conducted a study where he wanted to determine the effect of sexual intercourse on cervical status he did not find a significant association. He used a weekly Bishop score as a method of evaluation of the cervix and found no significant difference in scores in those women who had sexual intercourse and those who did not.

A Brustman et al. study [57] investigated changes in the pattern of uterine contractility before, between and after sexual intercourse. The study population consisted of 30 pregnant subjects. In group 1 were 15 women treated for an episode of preterm labour with intravenous and oral tocolysis in this pregnancy, and in group 2 were low-risk volunteers. Using home uterine tocodynamometric systems they monitored uterine contractility for three 60-minute time periods related to coitus. A significant increase in uterine contractility in the immediate postcoital period was observed for the high-risk women, but not for the controls. This increased uterine activity subsided spontaneously within two to three hours, returning to baseline. A small-scale experimental study of three normal gravid women between 28 and 38 weeks of pregnancy was performed by Chayen et al. [58] where they measured uterine contractility and foetal heart rate during sexual intercourse. Baseline traces were obtained 20 minutes before coitus. Increased uterine activity and a variety of foetal heart changes were seen in most (four out of 13 recordings) instances immediately following orgasm.

There are a variety of studies that have aimed to find the connection between coitus and onset of labour, but most of them found no association. Perhaps one of the largest scale studies on the effect of sexual intercourse on labour was done by Mills et al. [59] in this study, data on 10 981 singleton, low-risk pregnancies were examined. The mothers were asked at time of delivery if there were any months when they did not have sexual intercourse during pregnancy. Pregnancy outcomes were determined by medical record review. Those having intercourse showed no increased risk of premature rupture of membranes, low birthweight or perinatal death at any gestational age. Women abstaining from intercourse had more unfavourable outcomes in the seventh and eighth months, but these differences were almost eliminated by adjustment for maternal age. Preterm delivery was no more frequent in those having intercourse than in those abstaining. Chiong Tan et al. [60] wanted to determine coital incidence at term and to estimate its effect on labour onset and mode of delivery. They analysed 200 healthy women with uncomplicated pregnancies who kept a diary of coital activity from 36 weeks of gestation until birth and answered a short questionnaire. Reported sexual intercourse at term was influenced by a woman's perception of coital safety, her ethnicity, and her partner's age. Coitus at term had no significant effect on operative delivery. Reported sexual intercourse at term was associated with earlier onset of labour and reduced requirement for labour induction at 41 weeks. A year later, Chiong Tan et al. [61] estimated the effect of coitus on the onset of labour. A total of 102 women with a non-urgent labour induction at term were recruited. Women randomly assigned to the advised-coitus group were encouraged to have sex to promote the onset of labour. The control group was neither encouraged nor discouraged regarding coitus. Participants kept a coital and orgasm diary until delivery, and standard obstetric care was provided to both groups. Primary outcomes were reported for coitus and spontaneous labour. Secondary outcomes included reported orgasms, initial Bishop score at the admission for induction, preterm rupture of membranes, use of dinoprostone, oxytocin, or epidural, meconium-stained amniotic fluid, caesarean delivery, maternal fever, and neonatal morbidity. Spontaneous labour rate was no different [55.6% compared with 52.0%). Caesarean delivery rate and neonatal and other secondary outcomes were also not different. Among women scheduled for labour induction who were advised to have sex, the increase in sexual activity did not increase the rate of spontaneous labour. In 2009 Chiong Tan et al. [62] tried to evaluate the relationship of reported coitus and orgasm with spontaneous labour at term. Women at term scheduled for non-urgent labour induction were asked to keep a coitus and orgasm diary. These women were recruited for a randomized trial on the effect of coitus to promote spontaneous labour as mentioned above. Women who reported coitus were less likely to go into spontaneous labour prior to their scheduled labour induction. Reported coitus and orgasm were not associated with adverse pregnancy outcomes.

Premature rupture of membranes (PROM) as a possible adverse pregnancy outcome due to coitus was also researched. Ekwo et al. [63] tested the hypothesis that during late pregnancy sexual behaviours including sexual positioning related to the occurrence of premature rupture of membranes. They included women aged 15 to 45 years having preterm premature rupture of membranes, term premature rupture of membranes, or preterm delivery without premature rupture of membranes and were matched singly by age, race, and parity to control women who delivered term infants. Information about six sexual activities, obstetric history, cervical infections, smoking during pregnancy, and sociodemographic information was obtained by interview. Their results showed that only the male superior position was significantly associated with preterm premature rupture of membranes and preterm delivery without premature rupture of membranes after confounding variables were controlled for. No sexual positioning or sexual activities related significantly to term premature rupture of membranes. Oboro et al. [64] researched the possibility of sexual activity causing the PROM in Nigeria. They studied 97 consecutive patients [194 including control group without PROM) with a singleton normal pregnancy who had spontaneous prelabour rupture of foetal membranes. All patients were between 20 and 40 years of age, and at not less than 28 weeks of gestation at delivery. After delivery, a self-administered questionnaire with 17 items was offered to the women. Their findings did not show greater sexual activity in patients who had PROM. Coital frequency decreased progressively towards the end of pregnancy and was similar in both groups. There were no significant differences in the frequency of orgasmic coitus between the two groups. As seen so far, no study confirming sexual activity is associated with premature rupture of membranes.

Nipple stimulation has also been researched as a method of natural inducing labour. It has been reported to encourage cervical ripening, with an increase in the number of women spontaneously starting in labour [65, 66]. The stimulation was, for the purpose of the study, used three hours per day for three days, and this is barely considered to be natural.

There seems to be no scientifically proven natural sexual methods of induction of labour. However, a quest to find them still exists, probably because medical methods of induction are invasive, require hospitalization and include vaginally administered prostaglandins or amniotomy with or without intravenous oxytocin administration. Besides this, they are too often used without any strong medical justification.

Key points:

- Sex is generally considered safe late in pregnancy, at term.
- F and E series prostaglandins play an important role in ripening the cervix and contribute to contractibility of the uterus.
- Increased uterine activity and a variety of foetal heart changes were observed immediately following maternal orgasm.
- Sexual activity at term is not associated with increased risk of premature rupture of membranes.
- Sexual activity at term is not associated with increased risk of premature birth.

4. Sexual activity after childbirth

The first months after birth can have a great impact on women's sexual lives [21]. Postpartum sexual functioning is influenced by many factors, by significant anatomical changes, hormonal milieu, by the relationship between the partners, the way the family and support is structured and many other things. Sexual health after birth in the past did not receive enough attention from healthcare providers, but recent literature provides emerging attention to this aspect of postpartum care [67]. It is almost impossible to say what optimal sexual function after birth is. Connoly et al. [68] based on the results of their longitudinal prospective study, claim that within three months of birth 80-93% of women resume sexual intercourse, with sexual problems dissolving typically within one year postpartum. Luire et al. [69] speak of three mechanisms which may contribute to sexual dysfunction afterbirth: dyspareunia, birth canal injury and overall general health of mother. Much more precisely von Sydow [7] divides factors associated with decreased sexual interest, activity and enjoyment and increased sexual problems during postpartum (see Table 2]. She sees possible sexual dysfunction as a complex interplay by biomedical, psychosocial, couple/relationship factors as well as attributes of the baby and mother-child relationship.

http://dx.doi.org/10.5772/59496

Biomedical factors:
• Degree of perineal birth trauma. • Assisted vaginal delivery. • Tiredness. • Kegel exercise not performed. • No reliable method of contraception.
Psychosocial factors:
• Mental symptoms (depressed mood, emotional liability). • Prepregnancy sexual history and sexual symptoms. • Poor childhood relationship with father.
Couple relationship factors:
• Low relationship satisfaction.
Attributes of the baby and mother-child relationship:
• Male babies: mothers of boys are perceived less tender by their partners as mother of girls. • Mothers with rigid and overprotective relationship to their baby. • Breastfeeding.

Table 2. Factors associated with sexual dysfunction [7]

Postpartum sexual dysfunction (including dyspareunia) is identified in 41-83% of women at two to three months postpartum [70]. Leeman [70] describes that sexual dysfunction can be primary, indicating lifelong dysfunction, or secondary, indicating a change in function. Although many women are reporting more than one sexual disorder at a time, most common is lack of desire or sexual interest [70].

4.1. Physical changes associated with birth

Physical changes associated with birth and postpartum may influence a woman's sexuality. Following normal spontaneous delivery the vagina is wider and can be bruised and swollen [53]. The hormonal milieu causes the vaginal wall to lubricate poorly. This usually causes vaginal soreness during intercourse [71]. This is caused by lower levels of oestrogen. For breastfeeding mothers, levels of oestrogen are lower than in those who are not breastfeeding, and the dryness can be more marked. Experiencing discomfort with sexual intercourse is likely to discourage women from desiring sexual intercourse on subsequent occasions and reduce their sexual satisfaction [72].

Perineal or genital tract trauma is associated with postpartum dyspareunia. The research about whether this perineal trauma negatively impacts on sexual health after childbirth carries confounded results due to a variety of factors such as a postpartum timeframe, elective versus restrictive episiotomy and suturing or not suturing [73]. Compared to women who had normal spontaneous deliveries, women with episiotomies complained of increased perineal pain, decreased sexual satisfaction and a delay in restoring sexuality after birth [74-77]. Rathfish et al. [78] report that women who had episiotomy or second degree tear had lower levels of arousal, orgasm and sexual satisfaction and dyspareunia at three months postpartum, compared to women with an intact perineum. Leeman et al. [79] compared the postpartum pelvic floor function of women with sutured second-degree perineal lacerations, unsutured second-degree perineal lacerations, and an intact perineum. At 12 weeks postpartum, no differences were noted between groups regarding complaints of urinary or anal incontinence, sexual inactivity, or sexual function. However, in the same study Rodgers et al. [80] assessed sexual function at three months postpartum in women with genital trauma at birth. Trauma was categorized into minor trauma (no trauma or first-degree perineal or other trauma that was not sutured) or major trauma (second-, third-, or fourth-degree lacerations or any trauma that required suturing). Women who underwent episiotomy or operative delivery were excluded. Both trauma groups were equally likely to be sexually active. Significant differences were demonstrated: women with major trauma reported less desire to be held, touched, and stroked by their partner than women with minor trauma, and women who required perineal suturing reported lower Intimate Relationship Scale scores than women who did not require suturing.

4.2. The mode of delivery

There is extensive literature that has researched modes of delivery and their impact on sexual function after birth. The evidence does suggest a strong link between operative vaginal delivery and impaired sexuality after birth [81–87]. The somewhat protective role of caesarean sections has been noted as contributing to an early reestablishment of sexuality [21]. Johnsson [21] says that potential mechanisms may include minimal pudendal nerve injury, less trauma to the pelvic floor by the process of labour and the elimination of lacerations, episiotomy and diminished pain postpartum. There are some studies that have demonstrated this [87, 88] and some that have not [89]. Trauma to the pudendal nerve, however, has been demonstrated after vaginal delivery [21]. The main symptom of pudendal nerve trauma is pain in one or more of the areas innervated by the pudendal nerve or one of its branches. These areas include the rectum, anus, urethra, perineum, and genital area. In women this includes the clitoris, mons pubis, vulva, the lower 1/3 of the vagina, and labia [57]. Intrapartum pudendal nerve injury may be caused by compression of the foetal head. Stretch injury of pudendal nerve may be caused by a prolonged second stage of labour, operative delivery and large foetus [21]. Recovery usually takes two to six months [90].

Hicks et al. [91] performed a systematic review of the literature on selected postpartum sexual function outcomes as affected by caesarean, assisted vaginal, and spontaneous vaginal delivery. The studies all showed increased risks of delay in the resumption of intercourse, dyspareunia, sexual problems, or perineal pain associated with assisted vaginal delivery. Some studies showed no differences in sexual functioning between women with caesarean delivery and those with spontaneous vaginal delivery, whereas others reported less dyspareunia for women with caesarean delivery. A systematic review of the literature suggests an association between assisted vaginal delivery and some degree of sexual dysfunction. The reported associations between caesarean delivery and sexual dysfunction were inconsistent [91].

Safarinejad et al. [92] sought the relationship between mode of delivery and subsequent incidence of sexual dysfunction and impairment of quality of life in women and their husbands. A total of 912 pregnant women (mean age 26 +/- 2, range 21-32 years, parity I) and their husbands were recruited in this prospective study. The subjects were subdivided into five groups according to their mode of delivery, including: group A, spontaneous vaginal delivery (SVD) without injuries; group B, vaginal delivery with episiotomy (VDE) or perineal laceration; group C, operative vaginal delivery (OVD) (instrumental delivery), group D, planned caesarean section (PCS); and group E, emergency caesarean section (ECS). Of women in groups A, B, C, D, and E, 42.6%, 37.1%, 32.7%, 64.3%, and 38.3% resumed sexual intercourse (SI) within eight weeks of delivery. Women who experienced a PCS had the lowest pain scores, and women who had OVD had the highest pain scores at first SI (P = 0.001]. The research has shown that the quality of life parameters for PCS women were generally higher than for the other groups, and this concerns almost all categories. In healthy women with normal singleton pregnancies at term, instrumental deliveries are associated with the highest and PCS associated with the lowest rate of long-term maternal and paternal sexual dysfunction [92]. Connolly et al. [69] on the other hand found no difference at three or six months postpartum in timing of reestablishment of sexuality, dyspareunia or achieving orgasm whether women had caesarean section or vaginal delivery. Additionally, no impact was found of panned mode of delivery (vaginal vs. caesarean) on satisfaction with sexual relationship two years postpartum [93] and six years postpartum [94].

4.3. Dyspareunia

A very important determinant of postpartum sexual function is perineal pain and resultant dyspareunia (painful sexual intercourse). Perineal pain after a laceration is the most common cause of dyspareunia [79]. Dyspareunia is reported by 41%-67% of women two to three months postpartum and strongly associated with degree of perineal trauma. It has been reported that episiotomy with or without operative delivery is associated with dyspareunia and that spontaneous second-degree tears cause less perineal pain than episiotomy [95]. Connolly et al. [69] conducted a study to evaluate the effects of pregnancy and childbirth on postpartum sexual function. A total of 150 women were enrolled. Questionnaires were completed regarding sexual function prior to pregnancy, at enrolment, and at two, six, 12, and 24 weeks postpartum. At six, 12, and 24 weeks postpartum, 57%, 82%, and 90% of the women had resumed intercourse. At similar postpartum timepoints, approximately 30 or 17% of women reported dyspareunia; less than 5% described the pain as major. Delivery mode and episiotomy were not associated with intercourse resumption or anorgasmia; dyspareunia was only associated with breastfeeding at 12 weeks. However, no association was found with mode of delivery or the use of episiotomy.

Signorello et al. [96] wanted to investigate the possible association between the occurrence or/ and persistence of dyspareunia after childbirth and mode of delivery. Research was carried out with a retrospective cohort design in three groups of primiparous women after vaginal birth: Group 1 (n = 211] had an intact perineum or first-degree perineal tear; group 2 (n = 336] had second-degree perineal trauma; group 3 (n = 68] had third- or fourth-degree perineal trauma. At six months postpartum about one quarter of all primiparous women reported lessened sexual sensation, worsened sexual satisfaction, and less ability to achieve orgasm, as compared with these parameters before they gave birth. At three and six months postpartum, 41% and 22%, respectively, reported dyspareunia. Women with second-degree perineal trauma were 80% more likely and those with third- or fourth-degree perineal trauma were 270% more likely to report dyspareunia at three months postpartum. At six months postpartum, the use of vacuum extraction or forceps was significantly associated with dyspareunia, and women who breastfed were four times as likely to report dyspareunia as those who did not breastfeed. Women whose infants were delivered over an intact perineum reported the best outcomes overall, whereas perineal trauma and the use of obstetric instrumentation were factors related to the frequency or severity of postpartum dyspareunia [96]. These results were recently confirmed by Baksu et al. [97] who evaluated the effect of mode of delivery on postpartum sexual functioning in primiparous women. A total of 248 primiparous women were recruited into this study. Women who delivered vaginally and had mediolateral episiotomy reported significantly higher pain between six months postpartum than women with caesarean or spontaneous delivery. Not only pain, but also other important aspects of sexual function, such as arousal, lubrication, orgasm, and satisfaction were also affected by performing mediolateral episiotomy during vaginal delivery, well beyond the puerperal period. Concerning these effects, the authors recommended a policy of restricting mediolateral episiotomy.

It is seen from these study results that dyspareunia is mostly related to mode of delivery and problems that originate from that, and it is important that healthcare providers have knowledge of altered sexual life due to dyspareunia. The care they offer should be evidence-based and sensitive. Studies that have examined obstetricians' personal preferences toward delivery have indicated the major reason for avoiding vaginal delivery to be a fear of childbirth and concern for postpartum sexual health [21]. Caesarean delivery, as mentioned, appears to decrease the incidence of dyspareunia in the first three to six months postpartum, but has no effect beyond that frame. Despite the fact that some might see a caesarean section as a preventive measure for postpartum dyspareunia, studies have not confirmed this, and the fact that it is a major operation with possible serious side effects still remains.

4.4. Pelvic floor dysfunction

The pelvic floor is formed by the soft tissues that fill the outlet of the pelvis, and the most important of these is the strong diaphragm of muscle slung like a hammock from the walls of the pelvis, through it pass the urethra, the vagina and the anal canal [54, p. 107]. Pelvic floor dysfunction means weakened pelvic floor muscles cause the internal organs not to be fully supported and can this lead to difficulties in controlling the release of urine or faeces.

Studies suggest that vaginal delivery is associated with a higher rate of urinary of faecal incontinence than women who have undergone caesarean delivery [98-99]. It has to be noticed that none of the studies differentiate between an emergency caesarean section or planned caesarean section, or perhaps the length of the second stage in normal spontaneous delivery, which would be of great importance to the rate of urinary of faecal incontinence. It is also important, however, to address this issue due to the fact that urinary and faecal incontinence have a great impact on impaired sexual life and therefore quality of life postpartum [100].

4.5. Breastfeeding

There is quite strong evidence that suggests that breastfeeding reduces women's sexual desire and frequency of intercourse in postpartum [101-102]. Breastfeeding mothers have high levels of prolactin, which are maintained by babies' suckling. These high prolactin levels suppress ovarian oestrogen production, which results in reduced vaginal lubrication in response to sexual stimulation [54]. On the other hand, oxytocin release with breastfeeding causes milk ejection and appears to have positive effect on mood. Avery et al. [103] found that breastfeeding caused sexual arousal. The investigators used a descriptive design, analysing data from the 576 primiparous breastfeeding women who, as part of a larger study, completed the Breastfeeding and Sexuality Tool at the time of complete weaning. The women were from a large, private hospital in urban Minnesota. Subjects completed initial questionnaires during postpartum hospitalization. Follow-up data were collected by phone at one, three, six and 12 months postpartum. Those who had not been weaned by 12 months were followed every three months until complete weaning was reported. Overall, women perceived that breastfeeding had a slightly negative impact on the physiological aspects of sexuality, but did not greatly affect the woman's sexual relationship with her partner. In addition, breastfeeding mothers perceived their partners' attitudes towards breastfeeding and sexuality as slightly positive, and did not worry that sexual activity would harm their milk supply or their ability to nurse. Breastfeeding caused arousal frequently for 16.7% of women and infrequently for 23.7% of women. Quite different results came from another study where breastfeeding women have reported experiencing vaginal dryness, dyspareunia, increased nipple sensitivity, leaking milk and decreased arousal [67]. Barrett et al. [104] identify in their study a lack of interest in sexual activity at two months after birth that is strongly associated with breastfeeding, and dyspareunia is reported to persist for up to six months in some breastfeeding women. As seen, there are conflicting data as to whether breastfeeding increases or decreases sexual arousal. Some women also report physical contact with their infant as fulfilling a desire for contact that may otherwise be fulfilled with their partners; moreover, experienced breastfeeders report less of a reduction in sexual frequency than first-time breastfeeders [104].

4.6. Fatigue

Fatigue is a key component in the experience of parenting, and one of the most common problems women experience postpartum [6]. In three different studies [105-107] 62% of women report fatigue to interfere with their sexual life four months postpartum. Byrd et al. [108] state that fatigue accounted for considerable variability in postpartum women's decreased sexual desire. Despite this, fatigue is rarely studied as an independent variable.

4.7. Some psychological issues

There are many psychological issues that could affect postpartum sexuality such as stress and depression, relationship factors, perceived motherhood and others. There are few studies that research the relationship between depression and sexual activity postpartum. Morof et al. [109] researched the sexual health experiences of depressed and nondepressed postnatal women within a six-month postnatal period. Sexual health problems were common after childbirth in both depressed and nondepressed group; however, depressed women were less likely to have resumed intercourse at six months and more likely to report sexual health problems. Depressed women have decreased sexual desire, which may contribute to increased postpartum sexual function [21]. Research surrounding relationship satisfaction postpartum consistently demonstrates associations between partnership dissatisfaction and reduction in sexual activity, desire and enjoyment [104], while high-level support from a partner has been associated with greater sexual enjoyment [21]. For most women motherhood is a positive experience [110], but some might find negative aspects, such as a lack of uninterrupted time to pursue personal interests, quite disturbing [111]. There is some empirical evidence that such difficulties have an impact on sexual life; Pertot [112] found some evidence to suggest that problems in women's postpartum sexual responsiveness might be associated with difficulties with their mother role. Positive body image is generally thought to contribute to postpartum sexuality in women, though the associations are ambiguous [104]. It is already known that women who are satisfied with the way they look enjoy more sexually [7], but the fact that below 30% of women are satisfied with the way they look still remains [104]. Additionally, postpartum, besides adaptation to the role of mother, a lot of physical changes occur, weight needs some time to drop, breasts are changing, women might have abdominal striae or varicose veins, they might be lacking sleep and be experiencing many other things that potentially influence her body image in a negative way. Olsson et al. [113] conducted a series of focus group interviews to determine how some women experienced their sexual life with their partner after giving birth. Four themes were identified: body image after childbirth, how sexual patterns are altered following new stresses of family life, discordance of sexual desire with partners, and the necessity for reassurance. The women did not feel comfortable with the physical changes that had taken place and their body image. Childbirth meant less sleep and less free time; consequently, instead of having sex, women wanted to sleep or have time for themselves, and that led to a changed sex pattern. Discordance of sexual desire with the partner was a problem but most of the women expressed confidence that their sexual desire would return shortly. Reassurance and confirmation that they were physically acceptable and back to normal was essential. New mothers are concerned with their body image and their ability to adapt to parenting [113]. It seems that women need reassurance from healthcare professionals that their physical, psychological and bodily changes are a normal part of their childbearing.

Some risk factors for altered sexual health postpartum were identified. There might also be cultural or societal aspects regarding resumption of sexual activity but which were not discussed in this subchapter. Recommendations for practice by healthcare providers will be given in the concluding chapter.

5. Conclusion

Sexuality of expectant parents is of great importance, from a medical and psychological point of view. Childbearing is a period of incredible change on many levels of health, and requires the adaptation of a couple to the new addition to their family. A couple might not be aware that these changes commonly occur, and a majority of women may not receive adequate information or anticipatory guidance on these alterations from their healthcare providers [21].

Although some aspects about communication with prospective parents were already given in the second subchapter, this conclusion will, rather than summarize what is already written, contain valuable information for healthcare providers about how to approach and talk to parents about their sexuality and how to minimize some of the adverse events in pregnancy and birth for optimizing the sexual health of a couple postpartum. Recommendations are summarized and adapted from two authors who are well known researchers and professionals on the selected topic; von Sydow [7] and Leeman et al. [79].

As mentioned in the second subchapter, healthcare professionals do not always have the awareness, knowledge and skills to deal with sexual problems. Many gynaecologists are uncertain about what sexual advice to give when problems occur in pregnancy [7] or are uncomfortable speaking about it with women [21]. However, since it is known by now that healthy sexuality in pregnancy is a key stage in the evolution of being a parent [44], healthcare providers should keep open conversations about this throughout the duration of their care.

von Sydow [7] summarized recommendations for taking a sexual history and giving patients sexual advice. She believes that a partner should always be included in this conversation if possible. Healthcare providers have to ask open questions and listen to the answers.

Depending on what time a healthcare provider approaches couples the following information should be obtained:
• Pregnancy: the current emotional, marital and sexual situation and the information needs of a woman and her partner • Postpartum: sexual interest, behaviour, coital pain or incontinence
Then, the healthcare provider should give the couple the information about normal changes during the transition into parenthood, for example:
• Pregnancy: some women have no sexual interest whereas in others sexual interest is intensified • Postpartum: Some mothers experience erotic feelings during breastfeeding, and some fathers are jealous about breastfeeding. Vaginal dryness might be associated with breastfeeding.
• Acknowledge women's and partners fears and uncertainties and respect the inner limitations that they probably have. • Give technical advice about the range of sexual options; tenderness, non-coital sexual activities, alternative coital positions... • Instruct the patient in self-help: post birth self-inspection of vulva with a hand mirror, exercises... • Be sensitive to sexual and non-sexual domestic violence.

Table 3. Recommendations for taking a sexual history and giving a patient sexual advice in pregnancy or postpartum [7]

Research has shown [7] that couples wish to receive more information about bodily changes and sexuality postpartum, and that counselling has been helpful. Leeman et al. [79] divides a clinical approach for prevention, evaluation and treatment of postpartum sexual concerns into three parts based on prenatal care, postpartum and postnatal care (see Table 4].

Prenatal Care
• Determine whether dysfunction was present before pregnancy. • Discuss changes in anatomy, physiology, and sexual function that commonly occur during pregnancy. • Discuss the likely safety of continuing sexual activity throughout pregnancy for most women. • Evaluate presence of depression during pregnancy. • Discuss option of perineal massage to minimize perineal trauma and postpartum pain.
Intrapartum
• Judicious use of operative vaginal delivery and selection of vacuum rather than forceps will decrease the incidence of anal sphincter lacerations. • Limit the use of episiotomy. • Careful postpartum examination to increase the detection and repair of anal sphincter lacerations. • Repair perineal lacerations with synthetic absorbable suture. • Discuss perineal pain, dyspareunia, and initiation of postpartum sexual activity before hospital discharge.
Postpartum
• Assess sexual function and address concerns, including considering the use of a brief sexual function screening questionnaire. • Assess perineal repair if dyspareunia is present. • Assess for presence of urinary and anal incontinence symptoms. • Encourage vaginal lubricants, particularly in breastfeeding women with a physiologic hypoestrogenic state. • Consider alternative positions. • Assess for postpartum mood changes, adequate rest, and time for intimacy.

Table 4. Clinical approach for prevention, evaluation and treatment of postpartum sexual concerns Leeman et al. [79]

Leeman and his colleagues [79] have offered the possibility of perineal massage as an option to minimize perineal trauma and postpartum pain. There are also many other things we can advise women to practice in order to minimize the risk of birth injury or to prepare her body optimally. One of them is pelvic floor exercise, formerly known as Kegel exercise. Research shows that exercising the pelvic floor muscles during pregnancy makes it less likely that urinary incontinence will occur after birth [104]. Continuing these exercises after pregnancy can help to prevent long-term problems, such as prolapse. Both prolapse and urinary incontinence have a great impact on altered sexual life [21]. What seems to be missing from Leeman et al.'s [79] intrapartum list is also the way that the second stage is delivered, the use of unnecessary actions to speed the birth process and not letting the nature taking its course, which are all influences on birth outcomes that have an impact on pain and subsequently on sexual life postpartum. A study confirms that midwifery-led care is associated with low rates of episiotomy and operative delivery and very low rates of postpartum pain measured by a validated pain scale [114].

Optimal sexual health for women consists of a variety of physical and psychological factors, and open dialogue to encourage women to discuss these sensitive issues should be part of routine maternity care. Endocrine and psychosomatic factors as well as anatomical changes during pregnancy and the different forms of delivery may provoke female sexual dysfunction. Concerning sexual dysfunction after birth, almost 25% of women report sexual dysfunctions after birth such as low desire, dyspareunia, anoorgasmy and difficulty in lubrication, and many complain of more than one dysfunction. Leeman et al. [79] say that for many women the primary factors affecting the resumption of satisfying sexual activity postpartum relate not only to healing perineal trauma, vaginal dryness associated with lactation, or the effects of treatment for postpartum depression, but are dependent also on achieving an acceptable amount of rest and adequate time and physical space for intimacy. Although during antenatal visits healthcare providers have a tendency to avoid discussion of sexual problems, it is of great importance for couples to receive adequate information about the reduction of sexual intercourse, decline of libido and desire and other possible effects commonly encountered during pregnancy and postpartum.

The literature on selected topics is, despite its abundance, limited to a longitudinal prospective methodological approach and validating assessment tools. It is critical in the future to establish high quality normative data on sexual functioning during childbearing. More research is also needed to evaluate male sexual function and the role of the partner in overall sexual health [21].

Author details

Teja Škodič Zakšek*

Address all correspondence to: teja.zaksek@zf.uni-lj.si

Ljubljana University, Health Faculty, Midwifery Department, Slovenia

References

[1] World health organsation. Defining sexual health: Report of a technical consultation on sexual health http://www.who.int/reproductivehealth/publications/sexual_health/defining_sexual_health.pdf (accessed 21 july 2014).

[2] Corbacioglu Esmer A, Akca A, Akbayir O, Goksedef BP, Bakir VL. Female sexual function and associated factors during pregnancy. Journal of Obstetrics and Gynaecology Research 2013; 39(6):1165-72.

[3] Jones C, Chan C, Farine D. Sex in pregnancy. Canadian Medical Association Journal 2011; 183(7):815-8.

[4] Foumane P, Mboudou ET, Sama JD, Baba S, Enama Mbatsogo BA, Ngwana L. Sexual activity during pregnancy and prognosis of labor in Cameroonian women: a cohort study. The Journal of Maternal-Fetal and Neonatal Medicine 2014; 27(13):1305-8

[5] Schaffir J. Sexual intercourse at term and onset of labor. Obstetrics & Gynecology 2006; 107(6):1310-4.

[6] Hipp LE, Low K, van Anders, SM. Exploring women's postpartum sexuality: social, psychological, relational, and birth-related contextual factors. Journal of Sexual Medicine 2012; 9: 2330-2341.

[7] von Sydow. Sexuality in Pregnancy and the Postpartum Period. In: Reece EA, Hobbins JC. (3 ed) Clinical Obstetrics: The Fetus & Mother. Oxford: Blackwell Publishing Ltd; 2007. p1016-1021.

[8] Pauleta JR, Pereira NM, Graca LM. Sexuality during Pregnancy. Australian and New Zealand Journal of Obstetrics and Gynaecology 2010;18(2): 114-117.

[9] Tosun Güleroğlu F, Gördeles Beşer N. Evaluation of sexual functions of the pregnant women. The Journal of Sexual Medicine 2014;11(1):146-53.

[10] Chang SR, Chang TC, Chen KH, Lin HH. Developing and validating a Taiwan version of the female sexual Function index for pregnant women. The Journal of Sexual Medicine 2009; 6(6):1609-1616.

[11] Naim M, Bhutto E. Sexuality during pregnancy in Pakistani women. Journal of the Pakistan Medical Association 2000;50(1):38-44.

[12] Adinma JI. Sexuality in Nigerian pregnant women: perceptions and practice. Australian and New Zealand Journal of Obstetrics and Gynaecology 1995;35(3):290-3.

[13] Shoja M. Changes in Sexual and Behavioral Relationships among Couples during Pregnancy. Qom University of Medical Sciences Journal 2011;5(3):23-35.

[14] Jamali S, Mosalanejad L. Sexual dysfnction in Iranian pregnant women. Iranian Journal of reproductive medicine 2013;11(6):479-86.

[15] Fok WY, Chan LY, Yuen PM. Sexual behavior and activity in Chinese pregnant women. *Acta* Obstetricia et Gynecologica Scandinavica 2005;84(10):934-8.

[16] Liu H, Hsu P, Chen K. Sexual activity during pregnancy in Taiwan: A Qualitative study. Sexual Medicine 2013;1:54-61.

[17] Malarewicz A, Szymkiewicz J, Rogala J. Sexuality of pregnant women. Ginekologia Polska 2006; 77(9):733-9.

[18] Isajeva J, Šilkūnas M, Drąsutienė GS, Bartkevičienė D. Features of the sexual life during pregnancy. Acta medica lituanica 2012;19(2): 67–74

[19] Kohsaka T, Min G, Lukas G, Trupin S, Campbell ET; Sherwood OD, Identification of specific relaxin binding cells in the human female. Biology of Reproduction 1998; 59:991-999.

[20] Johnson CE. Sexual health during pregnancy and the postpartum. The Journal of Sexual Medicine 2011; 8(5):1267-84.

[21] Warnock JK, Clayton A, Croft H, Segraves R, Biggs FC. Comparison of androgens in women with hypoactive sexual desire disorder: those on combined oral contraceptives (COCs) vs. those not on COCs. The Journal of Sexual Medicine 2006;3(5):878-82.

[22] Pessina MA, Hoyt RF Jr, Goldstein I, Traish AM. Differential regulation of the expression of estrogen, progesterone, and androgen receptors by sex steroid hormones in the vagina: immunohistochemical studies. The Journal of Sexual Medicine 2006;3(5):804-14.

[23] Stuckey BG. Female sexual function and dysfunction in the reproductive years: the influence of endogenous and exogenous sex hormones. The Journal of Sexual Medicine 2008;5(10):2282-90.

[24] Erol B, Sanli O, Korkmaz D, Seyhan A, Akman T, Kadioglu A. A cross-sectional study of female sexual function and dysfunction during pregnancy. The Journal of Sexual Medicine 2007;4:1381–1387.

[25] Thorne C, Stuckey B. Pelvic congestion syndrome presenting as persistent genital arousal: A case report journal of sexual medicine; 5(2):504-508.

[26] Lewis JA, Black JJ. Sexuality in Women of Childbearing Age. The journal of perinatal education; 15(2): 29–35.

[27] Kitzinger S. Women's experience of sex. (1st ed). New York: Putnam;1983. p 54-56.

[28] Masters WH, Johnson VE. Human Sexual Response. (1st ed).Toronto: New York: Bantam Books, 1966 p 24-26.

[29] Guana-Trujillo B, Higgins PG. Sexual intercourse and pregnancy. Health Care for Women International 1987;8(5–6):339–348.

[30] Glowacka M, Rosen N, Chorney J, Snelgrove Clarke E, George RB. Prevalence and Predictors of Genito-Pelvic Pain in Pregnancy and Postpartum: The Prospective Impact of Fear Avoidance. The Journal of Sexual Medicine 2014; doi: 10.1111/jsm.12675.

[31] Chang SR, Chen KH, Lin HH, Lin MI, Chang TC, Lin WA. Association of mode of delivery with urinary incontinence and changes in urinary incontinence over the first year postpartum. Obstetrics & Gynecology 2014;123(3):568-77.

[32] Radoš SN, Vraneš HS, Šunjić M. Limited role of body satisfaction and body image self-consciousness in sexual frequency and satisfaction in pregnant women. The Journal of Sexual Medicine 2014;51(5):532-41.

[33] Cunningham FG, Wenstrom K, Hauth J, Leveno K, Gilstrap L. Williams Obstetrics. (21st ed). NY: McGraw-Hill Companies; 2001.

[34] Jones C, Chan C, Farine D. Sex in pregnancy. Canadian Medical Association Journal 2011; 183(7): 815–818.

[35] Timor-Tritsch IE, Yunis RA. Confirming the safety of transvaginal sonography in patients suspected of placenta previa. Journal of Obstetrics and Gynaecology 1993 ;81(5 (Pt 1)):742-4.

[36] Blanchard AC, Pastorek JG 2nd, Weeks T. Pelvic inflammatory disease during pregnancy. Southeren medical journal 1987;80(11):1363-5.

[37] Yip L, Sweeny PJ, Bock BF. Acute suppurative salpingitis with concomitant intrauterine pregnancy. The journal of reproductive medicine 2002;47(11):959-61.

[38] Lara-Torre E, Pinkerton JS. Viable intrauterine pregnancy with acute salpingitis progressing to septic abortion. A case report. Archives of Gynecology and Obstetrics 2004;269(3):219-20.

[39] Phupong V, Rungruxsirivorn T, Tantbirojn P, Triratanachat S, Vasuratna A. Infected endometrioma in pregnancy masquerading as acute appendicitis Archives of Gynecology and Obstetrics 2004;269(3):219-20.

[40] Taylor BD, Darville T, Haggerty CL. Does bacterial vaginosis cause pelvic inflammatory disease? Sexually Transmitted Disease 2013 ;40(2):117-22.

[41] Neilson JP, Mutambira M. Coitus, twin pregnancy, and preterm labor. American Journal of Obstetrics and Gynecology 1989;160(2):416-8.

[42] Stammler-Safar M, Ott J, Weber S, Krampl E. Sexual behaviour of women with twin pregnancies. Twin Research and Human Genetic 2010;13(4):383-8.

[43] Serati M, Salvatore S, Siesto G, Cattoni E, Zanirato M, Khullar V, Cromi A, Ghezzi F, Bolis P. Female sexual function during pregnancy and after childbirth. The Journal of Sexual Medicine 2010;7(8):2782-90.

[44] Polomeno V. Sex and Pregnancy: A Perinatal Educator's Guide. The Journal of Perinatal Education 2000;9(4):15-27.

[45] Belimac JG: Department of Health:Guidelines on the Management of Sexually-Transmitted Infections (STI) In Pregnancy http://www.doh.gov.ph/sites/default/files/STI_guidelines_1.pdf (accessed 21 july 2014).

[46] Foux R. Sex education in pregnancy: does it exist? A literature review. Sexual and Relationship Therapy 2008;23(3) 271-7.

[47] Sheryl Kingsberg Just ask! Talking to patients about sexual function. Sexuality, Reproduction and Menopause 2004;2(4): 199–203.

[48] King TL, Brucker MC, Kriebs JM, Fahey J, Gegor CL, Varney H. Varney's Midwifery. (4th ed)Burlington: Jones & Bartlett Learning; 2003.

[49] Gaskin IM. Birth Matters: A Midwife's Manifesta. (1st ed). NY: A seventh stories press;2011.

[50] Gaskin IM. Ina May's Guide to Childbirth. (1st ed). NY: Bantam book;2003.

[51] Gaskin IM. Spiritual Midwifery. (4th ed).Summertown:Book publishing company; 2002.

[52] Fraser DM, Cooper MA. Myles textbook for midwives. (14th ed) Edinburgh: Churchill Livingstone; 2003.

[53] Toth M, Rehnström J, Fuchs AR. Prostaglandins E and F in cervical mucus of pregnant women. American journal of perinatology 1989 ;6(2):142-4.

[54] O'Brien WF. The role of prostaglandins in labor and delivery.Clinics in perinatology 1995;22(4):973-84.

[55] Wein AJ, Kavoussi LR, Novick AC, Partin AW, Peters CA. Campbell-Walsh Urology (10th ed). NY:Elsevier;2012.

[56] Brustman LE, Raptoulis M, Langer O, Anyaegbunam A, Merkatz IR. Changes in the pattern of uterine contractility in relationship to coitus during pregnancies at low and high risk for preterm labor. Journal of Obstetrics and Gynaecology 1989;73(2): 166-8.

[57] Chayen B, Tejani N, Verma UL, Gordon G. Fetal heart rate changes and uterine activity during coitus. *Acta* Obstetricia et Gynecologica Scandinavica1986;65(8):853-5.

[58] Mills JL, Harlap S, Harley EE. Should coitus late in pregnancy be discouraged? Lancet 1981;2(8238):136-8.

[59] Tan PC, Andi A, Azmi N, Noraihan MN. Effect of coitus at term on length of gestation, induction of labor, and mode of delivery. Obstetrics and Gynaecology 2006;108(1):134-40.

[60] Tan PC, Yow CM, Omar SZ. Effect of coital activity on onset of labor in women scheduled for labor induction: a randomized controlled trial. Obstetrics and Gynaecology 2007;110(4):820-6.

[61] Tan PC, Yow CM, Omar SZ. Coitus and orgasm at term: effect on spontaneous labour and pregnancy outcome. Singapore Medical Journal 2009;50(11):1062-7.

[62] Ekwo EE, Gosselink CA, Woolson R, Moawad A, Long CR. Coitus late in pregnancy: risk of preterm rupture of amniotic sac membranes. 1993 ;168(1 Pt 1):22-31.

[63] Oboro VO, Tabowei TO, Bosah JO. Sexual activities in pregnancy and prelabour rupture of membranes. http://www.sexualhealthmatters.com/v3iss3/article2.html (accessed 21 july 2014).

[64] Salmon YM, Kee WH, Tan SL, Jen SW. Cervical ripening by breast stimulation. Obstetrics & Gynecology 1986;67:21–4.

[65] Elliott MD, Flaherty JF. The use of breast stimulation to prevent postdate pregnancy. American Journal of Obstetrics and Gynecology 1984;149:628–32.

[66] O'Malley D., Smith V. Altered sexual health after childbirth: part 1. The Practising Midwife 2013;16(1) 30-32.

[67] Connolly A., Thorp J., Pahel L. Effects of pregnancy and childbirth on postpartum sexual function: a longitudinal prospective study. International Urogynecology Journal and Pelvic Floor Dysfunction 2005;16(4) 263-267.

[68] Lurie S., Aizenberg M., Sulema V., Boaz M., Kovo M., Golan A., Sadan O. Sexual function after childbirth by the mode of delivery: a prospective study. Archives of Gynecology and Obstetrics 2013;288(4) 785-792.

[69] Leeman L., Rogers R. Sex After Childbirth. Obstetrics & Gynecology 2012;119(3) 647-655.

[70] Ridley CM. Vulvodynia. Theory and management. Dermatologic Clinics 1998;16(4) 775-8, xiii.

[71] De Judicibus M., McCabe M. Psychological Factors and the Sexuality of Pregnant and Postpartum Women. Journal of Sex Research 2002;39(2) 94-103.

[72] O'Malley D., Smith V. Altered sexual health after childbirth: part 2. The Practising Midwife 2013;16(2) 27-29. Dabiri F., Yabandeh AP., Shahi A., Kamjoo A., Teshnizi SH. The effect of mode of delivery on postpartum sexual functioning in primiparous women. Oman Medical Journal 2014;29(4) 276-9.

[73] Laganà AS., Burgio MA., Ciancimino L., Sicilia A., Pizzo A., Magno C., Butticè S., Triolo O. Evaluation of recovery and quality of sexual activity in women during postpartum in relation to the different mode of delivery: a retrospective analysis. Minerva Ginecologica 2014;66(3)

[74] Ejegård H., Ryding EL., Sjogren B. Sexuality after delivery with episiotomy: a long-term follow-up. Gynecologic and Obstetric Investigation 2008;66(1) 1-7.

[75] Woranitat W., Taneepanichskul S. Sexual function during the postpartum period. Journal of the Medical Association of Thailand 2007;90(9) 1744-8.

[76] Yıldız H.The Relation Between Prepregnancy Sexuality and Sexual Function During Pregnancy and the Postpartum Period: A Prospective Study. Journal of Sex & Marital Therapy. 2013 Oct 28. [Epub ahead of print]

[77] Rathfisch G., Dikencik BK., Kizilkaya Beji N., Comert N., Tekirdag Al., Kadioglu A. Effects of perineal trauma on postpartum sexual function. Journal of Advanced Nursing 2010;66(12) 2640-9.

[78] Leeman LM., Rogers RG., Greulich B., Albers LL. Do unsutured second-degree perineal lacerations affect postpartum functional outcomes? Journal of American Board of Family Medicine 2007;20(5) 451-7.

[79] Rodgers CS., Lang AJ., Twamley EW., Stein MB. Sexual trauma and pregnancy: a conceptual framework. Journal of Women's Health 2003;12(10) 961-70.

[80] Fehniger JE., Brown JS., Creasman JM., Van Den Eeden SK., Thom DH., Subak LL., Huang AJ. Childbirth and female sexual function later in life. Obstetrics & Gynecology 2013;122(5) 988-97.

[81] Buhling KJ., Schmidt S., Robinson JN., Klapp C., Siebert G., Dudenhausen JW. Rate of dyspareunia after delivery in primiparae according to mode of delivery. European Journal of Obstetrics & Gynecology and Reproductive Biology 2006;124(1) 42-6.

[82] Liebling RE., Swingler R., Patel RR., Verity L., Soothill PW., Murphy DJ. Pelvic floor morbidity up to one year after difficult instrumental delivery and cesarean section in the second stage of labor: a cohort study. American Journal of Obstetrics & Gynecology 2004;191(1) 4-10.

[83] Fallat ME., Weaver JM., Hertweck SP., Miller FB. Late follow-up and functional outcome after traumatic reproductive tract injuries in women. The American Journal of Surgery 1998;64(9) 858-61.

[84] McDonald EA., Brown SJ. Does method of birth make a difference to when women resume sex after childbirth? An International Journal of Obstetrics and Gynaecology 2013;120(7) 823-30.

[85] Woranitat W., Taneepanichskul S. Sexual function during the postpartum period. Journal of the Medical Association of Thailand 2007;90(9) 1744-8.

[86] Laganà AS, Burgio MA, Ciancimino L, Sicilia A, Pizzo A, Magno C, Butticè S, Triolo O. Evaluation of recovery and quality of sexual activity in women during postpartum in relation to the different mode of delivery: a retrospective analysis. Minerva Ginecol. 2014 [Epub ahead of print].

[87] Fauconnier A., Goltzene A., Issartel F., Janse-Marec J., Blondel B., Fritel X. Late postpartum dyspareunia: does delivery play a role? Progrès en Urologie 2012;22(4) 225-32.

[88] da Silva FM, de Oliveira SM, Bick D, Osava RH, Tuesta EF, Riesco ML. 89 Risk factors for birth-related perineal trauma: a cross-sectional study in a birth centre. Journal of Clinical Nursing 2012;21(15-16) 2209-18.

[89] Chaliha C. Postpartum pelvic floor trauma. Current Opinion in Obstetrics and Gynecology 2009;21(6) 474-9.

[90] Hicks TL., Goodall SF., Quattrone EM., Lydon-Rochelle MT. Postpartum sexual functioning and method of delivery: summary of the evidence. Journal of Midwifery & Women's Health 2004;49(5) 430-6.

[91] Safarinejad MR., Kolahi AA., Hosseini L. The effect of the mode of delivery on the quality of life, sexual function, and sexual satisfaction in primiparous women and their husbands. The Journal of Sexual Medicine 2009;6(6) 1645-67.

[92] Hannah ME, Whyte H, Hannah WJ, Hewson S, Amankwah K, Cheng M, Gafni A, Guselle P, Helewa M, Hodnett ED, Hutton E, Kung R, McKay D, Ross S, Saigal S,

Willan A; Term Breech Trial Collaborative Group. Maternal outcomes at 2 years after planned cesarean section versus planned vaginal birth for breech presentation at term: the international randomized Term Breech Trial.

[93] American Journal of Obstetrics & Gynecology 2004;191(3) 917-27.

[94] Dean N, Wilson D, Herbison P, Glazener C, Aung T, Macarthur C. Sexual function, delivery mode history, pelvic floor muscle exercises and incontinence: a cross-sectional study six years post-partum. Australian and New Zealand Journal of Obstetrics and Gynaecology 2008;48(3) 302-11.

[95] Yeniel AO, Petri E. Pregnancy, childbirth, and sexual function: perceptions and facts. International Urogynecology Journal 2014;25(1) 5-14.

[96] Signorello LB, Harlow BL, Chekos AK, Repke JT. Postpartum sexual functioning and its relationship to perineal trauma: a retrospective cohort study of primiparous women. American Journal of Obstetrics & Gynecology 2001;184(5) 881-8.

[97] Baksu B, Davas I, Agar E, Akyol A, Varolan A. The effect of mode of delivery on postpartum sexual functioning in primiparous women. International Urogynecology Journal and Pelvic Floor Dysfunction 2007;18(4) 401-6.

[98] Gyhagen M, Bullarbo M, Nielsen TF, Milsom I. Faecal incontinence 20 years after one birth: a comparison between vaginal delivery and caesarean section. International Urogynecology Journal 2014;25(10) 1411-8.

[99] Li WY, Liabsuetrakul T, Stray-Pedersen B. Effect of mode of delivery on perceived risks of maternal health outcomes among expectant parents: a cohort study in Beijing, China. BMC Pregnancy and Childbirth 2014;14(1) 12.

[100] Connolly A, Thorp J, Pahel L. Effects of pregnancy and childbirth on postpartum sexual function: a longitudinal prospective study. International Urogynecology Journal and Pelvic Floor Dysfunction 2005;16(4) 263-7.

[101] van Anders SM, Hipp LE, Kane Low L. Exploring co-parent experiences of sexuality in the first 3 months after birth. The Journal of Sexual Medicine 2013;10(8) 1988-99.

[102] Abdool Z, Thakar R, Sultan AH. Postpartum female sexual function. European Journal of Obstetrics & Gynecology and Reproductive Biology 2009;145(2) 133-7.

[103] Avery MD, Duckett L, Frantzich CR. The Experience of Sexuality During Breastfeeding amound Primiparous Women. Journal of Midwifery and Women's Health 200;45(3) 227-237.

[104] Barrett G, Peacock J, Victor CR, Manyonda I. Cesarean section and postnatal sexual health. Birth 2005;32(4) 306-11.

[105] Fischman SH, Rankin EA, Soeken KL, Lenz ER. Changes in sexual relationships in postpartum couples. Journal of Obstetric, Gynecologic, & Neonatal Nursing 1986;15(1) 58–63.

[106] Ahlborg T, Strandmark M, Dahlof LG. First-time parents' sexual relationships. Scandinavian Journal of Sexology 2000;3 127–39.

[107] Ahlborg T, Dahlof L, Hallberg LR. Quality of intimate and sexual relationship in first-time parents six months after delivery. Journal of Sex Research 2005;42(2) 167–74

[108] Byrd JE, Hyde JS, Delamater JD, Plant EA. Sexuality during pregnancy and the year postpartum. The journal of family practice1998; 47 (4): 305-308.

[109] Morof D, Barrett G, Peacock J, Victor CR, Manyonda I. Postnatal depression and sexual health after childbirth.Obstetrics and Gynecology 2003;102(6) 1318-1325.

[110] Anwar E, Stanistreet D. 'It has not ruined my life; it has made my life better': a qualitative investigation of the experiences and future aspirations of young mothers from the North West of England. Journal of Public Health: Oxford Journals 2014 Jul 6. pii: fdu045.

[111] Hoffenaar PJ, van Balen F, Hermanns J. The Impact of Having a Baby on the Level and Content of Women's Well-Being. Social Indicators Research 2010;97(2) 279-295.

[112] Pertot S. Postpartum loss of sexual desire and enjoyment. Australian Journal of Psychology 1981;33(1) 11–18.

[113] Olsson A, Lundqvist M, Faxelid E, Nissen E. Women's thoughts about sexual life after childbirth: focus group discussions with women after childbirth. Scandinavian Journal of Caring Sciences 2005;19(4) 381-7.

[114] Leeman L, Fullilove AM, Borders N, Manocchio R, Albers LL, Rogers RG. Postpartum perineal pain in a low episiotomy setting: association with severity of genital trauma, labor care, and birth variables. Birth 2009;36(4) 283-8.

Chapter 6

The Experience of Pregnancy, Childbirth and Motherhood in Women with a History of Sexual Abuse

Tanja Repič Slavič and Christian Gostečnik

Additional information is available at the end of the chapter

http://dx.doi.org/10.5772/59085

1. Introduction

Sexual abuse is a traumatic experience that marks a person for the rest of their life and has numerous consequences. Some effects may manifest immediately, others only years afterwards. The trauma may even be transferred to the following generations. The purpose of this paper is to present the *theory* and existing *research* in the field of sexual abuse. It also provides an exploration of clinical practice, with descriptions of group therapy cases. It presents the findings of three therapy groups for sexually abused women. Each group included ten participants who met with a family therapist and co-therapist for one year. On the basis of *analysing the content* of their diaries, we describe the therapist's notes and supervision notes (in line with the *grounded theory* method) regarding the most typical experiences relating to pregnancy, childbirth and motherhood.

This paper begins with the definition of sexual abuse, its consequences and the survival methods most commonly used by the abused.

We continue by considering the impact of sexual abuse on the victim's experience of **pregnancy**, **childbirth** and **motherhood**.

During pregnancy, a woman's body is particularly sensitive. This is due to the many organ changes that effect her psychic and physical state. Research results show that, during pregnancy, a sexually abused woman has more health problems and is more frequently in conflict with her partner. Furthermore, she experiences higher levels of anxiety and fear, compared to those who have not been sexually abused.

During childbirth itself, a mother with a history of sexual abuse has more trust issues with the personnel. Moreover, during gynaecological examinations, she experiences flashbacks that subconsciously trigger her body's memory of the sexual abuse. During the contractions and pushing, when the woman in labour needs to co-operate most with the medical staff, her body or psyche can react by freezing, panicking or taking complete control. She is also more prone to a caesarean section and other complications.

These feelings and experiences are also often present *in motherhood*. Compared to a mother who has not been sexually abused, a mother with a history of sexual abuse experiences more feelings of guilt, troubles with breastfeeding and various fears.

We conclude this paper by expressing our hope that one can work through the trauma of sexual abuse and start living a full life. Clinical experiences have shown that a woman who resolves her trauma is much more relaxed and happy during pregnancy. She is calmer during childbirth and is a more compassionate mother, compared to a woman who does not resolve her trauma. After all, if the little girl survived the trauma when it happened, she can now survive as a grown woman - the abuse is **no longer** happening, it is only awakening.

2. Definition of sexual abuse

Sexual abuse is a traumatic experience involving an involuntary sexual contact between the abuser and the victim, with the intention of sexually arousing the perpetrator who transgresses all limits of human dignity [1]. The actions are not limited to a forced sexual intercourse but include a wide range of sexual behaviours, most commonly the following: exposing one's genitals, observing a child, using pornography, groping, masturbating in front of the victim or forcing the victim to masturbate while the offender watches, fellatio, cunnilingus, digital or object penetration of the anus or vagina, sodomy, etc. [2].

Clinical practice has shown that it is very difficult to predict what consequences a victim will experience. This is because they depend on several factors: the age and sex of the abused, the seriousness of the abuse, the relation between the victim and the offender (whether the offender is a family member or not, a known person, an unknown person, etc.), whether the child told anyone about the abuse and, if they did, what the response was and the duration of the abuse [3-6].

Many abused individuals are too focused on survival to notice how the abuse has effected them. Even worse, most do not even think that the effects and problems they experience could be related to sexual abuse. They are ashamed of what they did to survive, even though, in the given situation full of pain, that was the best possible solution. The most common kinds of behaviour that the abused adopt to survive are: derogation, rationalization, denial, forgetting and running away from reality (split, dissociation), constant control, hypervigilance, perfectionism, freezing, absentmindedness, busyness, escape, humour, lying and stealing, religious fanaticism, drug and alcohol abuse, overeating, engaging in unhealthy and risky sexuality, obsessive masturbating, etc. [7].

3. The consequences of sexual abuse

In general, it is difficult to say how sexual abuse impacts an abused person. This is because sexual abuse effects everything: self-confidence, sexuality, intimate relationships, parenthood, work, mental health, body, etc. Additionally, some consequences may be visible immediately, whilst others only come to light years after. They awaken in various situations reminiscent of the abuse. Recent studies have shown that they can even come to an intergenerational transmission of trauma. This means that the effects manifest in future generations, in children born after the trauma had already taken place (e.g., war veterans and their children and grandchildren) [8]. Sexual abuse has an impact on both the physical and the psychical area of human action, which strongly marks and changes a person's life. In most cases, the effects are long-term, extremely radical and harmful. More rarely, the effects can be short-term [7-10].

Short-term consequences: unwanted pregnancy, higher risk of sexually transmitted diseases, infertility, various gynaecological inflammations and pains in the lower abdomen, infections of the urinary bladder, abrasions and laceration on various parts of the body, bruises and redness, more frequent chronic somatic diseases, a negative attitude towards one's body, chronic fatigue and exhaustion, sleeping disorders, eating disorders, very painful menstruation, fear, apprehension and anxiety, troubles concentrating and thinking, emotional irritability and hypersensitivity, hate and aggression, promiscuous behaviour, etc.

Long-term consequences: many of the above also belong among the long-term consequences but the effects that most often come to light after many years, on the other hand, can sometimes appear soon after the abuse. The most frequent among them are: post-traumatic stress disorder, social phobias, fear and anxiety, guilt and shame, substance abuse and eating disorders, running away from home, depression, suicide, panic attacks, excessive distrust, troubles with interpersonal relationships, partner relations, infidelity and physical violence, sexual dysfunctions and other problems with sexuality, personality disorders and dissociations, likelihood of re-victimization, low self-esteem, sexualized behaviour in children, regression in behaviour, self-harming, etc.

4. The trauma of sexual abuse, body and health issues

Sexual abuse first occurs at a physical level. This is precisely why many victims of sexual abuse blame their bodies for having responded; for being attractive, small, vulnerable and susceptible to arousal and pleasure. They accuse themselves for even having bodily sensations. Thus, in some respects, relaxation can pose a subconscious risk of something bad happening. This is why victims feel it is safer to be alert and awake - a sexually abused child can never really relax. Many victims of sexual abuse experience their bodies as a burden and a nuisance. They do take it into account because, precisely when it should have defended itself, it ran away and betrayed them. Part of not paying heed to their bodily needs is not hearing the body. This also applies when people are ill; they hold in their urine because they want to finish a small task, they do not rest when it is high time for them to take a break, they go to extremes with eating and performing physical activities, they harm themselves, develop various forms of addiction, etc. [7].

It is often the case that medical examinations and tests do not explain the symptoms of a patient who has experienced a trauma. This does not mean that the patient does not suffer physical pain, only that the cause of the pain is psychosomatic. A traumatic experience effects not only the structure and functioning of the brain, but also the stability of one's psyche, one's thought processes and the health of one's body. In extreme cases, traumas can contribute substantially to psychiatric disorders [11]. Most of these patients seem demanding, afraid, uncertain and sometimes do not trust even those closest to them who ensure them that they are perfectly fine. Many suffer due to various medical symptoms, most often digestion problems, chronic fatigue and sleeping disorders. Scaer [11], who has worked as a doctor for many years and encountered various patients (those also injured in accidents or otherwise traumatized), believes that the various physical syndromes (pains) in traumatized people are more often a consequence of a certain experience, rather than a proven organ injury. *For example, stomach pain may be the result of a psychic distress experienced by a sexually abused person, rather than organ damage or food poisoning.* The trauma of sexual abuse can also impact neurological and hormonal (endocrinological) changes, the immune system, etc. A person's emotional state effects their physical wellbeing and health. There is an increasing number of scholars [11-13] who emphasize that the mind, brain and body are related. The brain operates and responds on the basis of stimuli that come from outside and inside the body. It compares present experiences with past ones. The body then responds to the brain's orders and changes, according to the stimuli and messages it receives through the brain. In view of all the stored memories, the mind then directs the body's behaviour and influences the content of the memories to be stored.

The above suggests that the atmosphere and emotional and physical states during the trauma are very closely connected to the operation and functioning of the brain. This then effects bodily changes, which also include diseases and one's health condition.

Studies in the field of health care and medicine [14] have generally shown that people who have been sexually abused in the past have more health issues, report more somatic symptoms and pains than people who are not victims of sexual abuse. They also report a greater degree of chronic diseases. The most common and most general are: gastrological diseases, stomach diseases (ulcer), respiratory disorders (e.g., asthma, bronchitis, emphysema), heart problems, hypertension, arthritis, diabetes and gynaecological problems. Gynaecological problems are most often related to the loss of the menstrual cycle or excessive bleeding, sexual dysfunctions, frequent pains in the lower abdomen (even when not during menstruation), frequent inflammation of genitalia and pains during sexual intercourse.

Golding [15] interviewed a group of women who were seeking help due to severe PMS. She found that 95% of the women reported that they had experienced at least one attempt of sexual abuse or were sexually abused. Furthermore, 81% of these women were raped.

Additionally, other studies [11,13] report chronic inflammation of the bladder and frequent and painful urinating - which only intensify during menstruation. Such studies estimate that 90% of women with a history of sexual abuse experience these problems.

It is precisely the above health issues that can lead to sexually abused women turning to pills and other medical devices.

In general, the trauma of sexual abuse can have a direct impact on the health of an abused person. This is because the victim could have been exposed to infection or even infected with an STD during the abuse itself. The abuse can also indirectly harm the victim's health. This is because abuse increases the probability of the abused person getting involved in abusive relationships. In this regard, relational family therapy explores the subconscious attractiveness of abuse or the loyalty to feelings reminiscent of abuse (disgust, shame, disdain, fear, etc.). The psyche subconsciously seeks such an atmosphere, with the hope that these effects will be resolved and that something new – non-abusive – will happen [16]. Studies have shown that people who have been raped are much more inclined to experience physical violence from a partner in a relationship, compared to people who have no history of rape [17]. It is this physical violence that increases the chances of those victims suffering more serious injuries.

Some scholars [18] have found that victims of sexual abuse can quickly begin to perceive their bodies as dysfunctional. This can lead to psychosomatic problems. Some victims also become preoccupied with every bodily change. Furthermore, upon every - even the slightest - sign of illness, they suffer real horrors as if they were seriously ill. The consequences of such psychical distresses and experiences are manifested physically, in organs. In other words, the psychical pain is transferred to the victim's body and her body tells her that there is something she can no longer endure.

All these physical signs are psychosomatic and can manifest in: headaches (only as tensions or migraines), sleeping disorders, appetite disorders, stomach problems, gynaecological issues (chronic pains in the lower abdomen, dyspareunia, vaginismus, non-specific vaginitis, menopausal disorders, etc.), asthmatic and heart problems, muscular tension, fainting fits, vertigo, fatigue, etc.

The same scholars explain psychosomatic problems that are consequences of sexual abuse with a chronically stimulated autonomic nervous system. This nervous system increases the release of hormones (epinephrine and cortisol). It is this constant releasing that has long-term effects on the body.

Sometimes, the psychosomatic problems in a certain part of the body injured during abuse appear much later, even after several years, e.g., pains in the jaw if the person had been raped orally. Additionally, problems may emerge that are more difficult to notice such as a weak immune system, susceptibility to colds and flu, chronic fatigue and exhaustion, etc. [7].

All the mentioned studies show that the trauma of sexual abuse is related to a higher degree of health problems. Such problems can also have an effect on pregnancy, which we will consider next.

5. Pregnancy and the history of sexual abuse

Body memory can awaken when a woman's body starts to change during pregnancy. When the pregnancy becomes visible, this can be a sign that the body is no longer untouchable, that someone has already crossed the "line". Thus, a woman's gestational belly becomes part of the public arena, where everybody notices and sees it. For a woman without a history of sexual abuse, this can be the most beautiful thing. However, for a woman who has been sexually abused, her body becoming more noticeable and different can be extremely distressing. This is particularly the case if, for years and years, she had hidden every bodily change caused by the sexual abuse - even if only in her feelings and experiences.

Some studies have shown that girls who have been sexually abused in childhood are three times more likely to get pregnant before the age of 18 years [19] than those who have not. Similarly, Saewyc et al. [20] argue that 60% of pregnant underage girls have been victims of sexual harassment, rape or attempted rape in their past. According to other studies, pregnancy (as a consequence of sexual abuse) occurs in 11% to 20% of girls. Furthermore, more than 96% of underage prostitutes who have run away from home have been victims of sexual abuse in their childhood [9].

A study on a sample of 3,128 sexually abused underage girls showed that they engage more often in sexually risky behaviour (promiscuity, prostitution and pornography – seeking contact through sexuality). This study also reported that, compared to girls who had not been sexual abused, these girls were more likely to have had intercourse by the age of 15 years and more than one sexual partner. They were also less likely to use birth control during intercourse. Additionally, they more often used alcohol or other substances before having sexual intercourse. Among others, the following variables strongly stood out in this study: lack of parental supervision, presence of physical abuse, higher levels of school absenteeism, less involvement in extracurricular activities and lower grades (in comparison to those who had not been sexually abused). The difference between the two groups was statistically significant. The study also demonstrated that underage girls with a history of either sexual or physical abuse were twice as likely to become pregnant as teenagers, compared to girls without such a history. If they had experienced both sexual and physical abuse, they were four times as likely to get pregnant [21].

Seng et al. [22] found that women who had experienced PTSD during pregnancy were more susceptible to a spontaneous abortion, ectopic pregnancy and hyperemesis. Other studies report that sexually abused women have a statistically significant higher number of complications during pregnancy. Among the most common are: bleeding, severe vomiting, x-ray or radiotherapy in the first semester, alcohol, smoking, medications, accidents, infectious diseases, threatened abortions with hospitalization and severe illness [23]. Some abused women report several health complications and a higher use of health care services during pregnancy. However, these women do not experience more obstetric complications during their pregnancies and deliveries [24].

Women with a history of sexual abuse **experience depression in the prenatal and the postnatal period much more often** than women who have not been sexually abused. In general, children whose mothers were depressed during pregnancy show changes in their neurological functioning. They are more withdrawn, irritable and inconsolable than children whose mothers were not depressed during pregnancy [25]. Prenatal depression can lead to deficient care during pregnancy and bad eating habits, as well as the abuse of various substances like tobacco, alcohol and illegal drugs.

Smoking can lead to spontaneous abortion, as well as increasing the risk of an enlarged thyroid gland in children, low body weight and deformation. It has been recorded that children whose mothers smoked heavily during pregnancy had lower mental abilities measured by the age of 19 months with the Bayley Scales of Infant Development [14]. The foetuses of women who chronically drank **alcohol** during pregnancy exhibited serious morphological (related to the form of the organism) and developmental abnormalities. Not all children exposed to alcohol during pregnancy suffer such serious conditions. However, there is a high probability that they will have neurological and cognitive disorders such as a lower reaction time and reduced attention spans.

Using illegal drugs during **pregnancy** is also problematic. Using **marihuana** during pregnancy can lead to a child having lower mental abilities, hyperactivity, impulsiveness, carelessness, inattention, delinquency and the externalizing of problems. **Cocaine abuse** during pregnancy is associated with a weakened, impaired processing of aural information, an increased risk of spontaneous abortion, premature labour pains, a stillborn child and microcephaly (the child having a small head). Heroine abuse and the use of other narcotics can cause a premature birth, the death of the foetus, the child's addiction, low body weight and cognitive and behavioural problems. **LSD and inhalants abuse** can be related to various deficits at birth [26].

In addition to drugs, women often silence their abused bodies with food. Waugh and Bulik [27] have found that women **with eating disorders during pregnancy** are more exposed to a caesarean section and have more problems in maintaining breastfeeding. Often, the disorders continue after the birth, leaving them at a high risk of developing postnatal depression.

Katarina Neff [28], a doula who has a lot of experience with pregnant women who have been sexually abused, believes that when a sexual abuse survivor with PTSD becomes pregnant, she may develop the following symptoms:

- Feelings of body betrayal
- Feelings of physical intrusion and invasion
- Flashbacks to the original abuse
- Depression
- Anxiety or panic
- Abuse memories resurfacing for the first time
- Antagonistic or hostile feelings toward the foetus
- Projecting feelings about the abuser onto the foetus
- Feelings of guilt (associated with her feelings)
- Feelings of shame (associated with body changes)

"Because birth is so different for every woman," comments Kristina, "women who have dealt with the same trauma may react in completely different ways and have completely different fears. Mostly, they are afraid of dealing with the first trauma again, regardless of if it was an abusive situation or a previous traumatic birth." There are some **specific fears that may manifest for a sexual abuse survivor with PTSD**, such as:

- Fear of the intensity of her feelings
- Fear that the child will be born deformed (like her)
- Fear that the child will be born dead (i.e., as punishment, wish fulfilment or self fulfilling prophesy)
- Fear of being an incompetent parent
- Fear of being an abusive parent

Sometimes the consequences of sexual abuse are not extensive or it does not seem that there are any. However, some women have been surprised and distressed by the feelings or memories that surface once they are pregnant, giving birth or mothering their child.

"Until I got pregnant, I had no problems or any difficult memories of the sexual abuse I had suffered in my childhood. It seemed to me that those who said it was a serious trauma exaggerated, since my life was quite okay. I don't know what happened afterwards, but I can't even describe the degree of worry, fear and anxiety I started experiencing after I got pregnant, especially after I started showing. A terrifying fear that I'd lose the child because my body was dirty due to the abuse and the child couldn't develop in such conditions...sudden and severe anxiety attacks because I no longer had control over my body, my weight, my belly, which kept growing..."

"My pregnancy was nothing special until the moment the child began kicking in my belly. I was overwhelmed by the uncontrollable feelings of panic. Once, I even had to go to the ER. I felt guilty because I just wanted to pull the child right out, since every movement that was not under my control unnerved me intensely. At moments, I even wished for the child to die so that the distress would stop but I knew that, then, another would begin. I was somewhat appeased by being told I was having a girl because I realized that a boy would obviously remind me too much of the perpetrator."

Clinical practice has shown that many pregnant women who have been sexually abused in the past often experience distress and new traumas in situations where women without a history of sexual abuse do not experience - or to a substantially smaller degree [29]. Even the usual gynaecological examinations can be very unpleasant due to the groping. In this case, it is very important that the gynaecologist is professional and sensitive. Nevertheless, when a woman is pregnant, carrying a developing and growing being, she is all the more sensitive to every touch and procedure related to her womanhood and her body [30].

"The visit to the gynaecologist reminds me very much of rape. You lie there like a victim, while he shines his light down there and touches you. I think that someone inserting their fingers in your vagina is a matter of sex and I can't imagine what else this action would be good for. I find the stirrups particularly horrible. But, on the other hand, I am also aroused. When I was at the gynaecologist's last year, I had the same feeling as after sex, only without the kissing and petting. Like a rape I myself wanted. I was

very much aroused when I went home and I was quite ashamed. I felt disgusted with myself and wished that someone would actually rape me. I'd pay him to go to bed with me and treat me really nastily, like his slave."

"It's the most horrible doctor's examination in the world. I go there when they send me the third invitation because I have to have regular check-ups. There I am, all stiff, keep my eyes closed and try to think of anything but this dreadful, humiliating, disgusting position I am in. The thought that I will have to go there almost every month when I'm pregnant makes me not want to ever get pregnant."

"What bothered me most was that some people touched my baby bump without permission. There were a few times when I had to leave the company and go to the toilet to vomit because I was so disgusted with the touching and, at the same time, angry with myself that I didn't draw the line and say I didn't like it."

Post-traumatic effects of sexual abuse can be a big problem for survivors and a source of great fear. This is due to the subconscious triggering of traumatic memories during pregnancy (prenatal care) and delivery (the experience of birth). Women may avoid necessary medical care because of these fears. Furthermore, they may be so devastated by their experiences that they have difficulty enjoying and caring for their newborns. With this in mind, it can be highly beneficial if the personnel (midwifes, doctors, doulas, etc.) that a woman encounters during pregnancy, childbirth and the postnatal period are acquainted with her trauma and react appropriately. This ensures an even greater feeling of safety and support for the traumatized woman. Compassion in such hard times accelerates the healing of the reawakened trauma. At the same time, unkindness, roughness and unprofessionalism re-traumatize the pregnant woman and cause her additional distress and pain [29].

6. Childbirth and the history of sexual abuse

It is normal for every pregnant woman to be afraid of giving birth. Evidence suggests that the fear of childbirth exists in a psychological domain of its own. For some women, the fear is of a very low level but for others, it can be extremely high [31]. Extreme fear of childbirth has been estimated to effect around 2.4% to 5% of pregnant women [32].

Numerous studies report that a great fear of childbirth is strongly related to negative sexual experiences in childhood and youth [33]. Fear may manifest itself by tearfulness, sleeplessness, nightmares, preoccupation with fear and the objects of fear, restlessness, nervousness and tachycardia. Fear of childbirth may include fear of any of the following: the labour and delivery process, labour pain, lack of care by health professionals, the health of the baby or mother, surgical procedures, damage to the vagina and perineum, loss of control, not performing well, panic attack, physical exposure, uncertainty about the process of labour and becoming a parent [34].

In addition to the fear of childbirth, other fears may also be present. For example, the fear of vaginal examinations, health professionals noticing that you are damaged even if you don't have scars, being touched without consent and loss of control.

A study that included 2,365 pregnant women reported that a history of sexual abuse significantly increased the risk of experiencing severe fear of childbirth among primiparae. Fear of childbirth among multiparae was most strongly associated with a negative birth experience [35].

Similar conclusions can be found in a study that included 1,452 pregnant women (at 18 weeks of gestation) and measured their fear of childbirth (with the W-DEQ questionnaire) and anxiety (with the STAI questionnaire). In this study, the serious fear of childbirth effected 5.5% of the women. The fear of childbirth is not associated with the mode of delivery. However, sexual or physical abuse in childhood is negatively associated with the mode of delivery [32]. A small number of studies have shown that a history of child abuse has a minimal effect on the complications of labour and mode of delivery [36]. Having said this, the majority of studies have shown the opposite [37-39].

An experimental study, which used the cold pressor test, has shown that women who are afraid of childbirth have a reduced level of pain tolerance during and after pregnancy, compared to women who are not afraid of childbirth [40]. Other studies have shown that pregnant women who fear childbirth are prone to report fear during the actual labour and postpartum [41]. Fear of childbirth has been associated with elective CS, hyperemises gravidarum, induction of labour, use of EDA and prolonged labour [42].

Compared to women with no history of sexual abuse, women with a history of sexual abuse are significantly more likely to be transferred to hospital due to complications. Furthermore, they use more medical pain relief, while primiparae are more likely to give birth with a CS [39].

A Norwegian study has shown that only half of women who report having an experience of physical and sexual abuse in childhood have a vaginal delivery without complications, as opposed to the 75% of non-abused women.

Similarly, a study in which 103 women were interviewed four weeks after giving birth showed that women who have been sexually abused are 12 times more likely to experience the childbirth event as traumatic [43].

The traumatic experience of childbirth is particularly associated with the subconscious awakening of the trauma of sexual abuse. This manifests through flashbacks and body memory. The most frequent triggers are vaginal examinations or other procedures (e.g., enema, shaving etc.). Additionally, pain during or after the childbirth itself can be a trigger, particularly in the woman's vagina, stomach, back, breasts or crotch. It is the person who a woman should trust the most during childbirth who can subconsciously remind her of the perpetrator who abused her trust as an authority figure (e.g., teacher, parent, stepfather, coach, priest, etc.). The woman then (re)experiences the feelings of powerlessness, humiliation, shame and horror [29].

During the labour pains, a woman with a history of sexual abuse can start to feel that she no longer controls her own body - just as she did during the abuse. This is why, for an abused woman, having no control often feels like she is no longer emotionally and physically safe and that something bad is about to happen. This is why she feels stronger and safer if things are structured – if she knows what will happen during labour, how it will roughly take place, what is normal and what she can expect. This information will help her to take a break from the constant control, worrying and waiting for what is to come. It is precisely these feelings that are very strongly related to the abuse they have suffered. Abuse teaches a person that it is "safer" to be constantly alert. Furthermore, the feeling of being endangered can lead to extreme behaviour, e.g., aggression, submission, rituals, constant crises, etc. [44].

"I had a problem with gynaecological examinations as long as I can remember. I can never completely relax. Having to spread my legs in front of a man that's not my partner instantly puts me in situations that I experienced as a child. I also faced traumas during childbirth. My subconscious spewed memories from the past and, even though I suffered painful labour pains, I couldn't help myself. The cervical exam...Horror, despair, panic, tears, anger...At that moment, I couldn't calm myself and make myself understand that the obstetrician was only going to examine me. Despite the labour pains and big belly, I lifted my backside from the bed and sought refuge at the wall. My husband and the nurses tried to calm me down, but I didn't care. The simple fact that someone wanted to examine me in the middle of my labour pains seemed extremely intrusive and horrible!"

During the sexual abuse of their bodies, some women are threatened. This can be not only verbally and psychically, but also physically (e.g., with a weapon). *"The labour pains intensified so quickly that I felt the gradual loss of control. I became more and more afraid. The pains got stronger and more intense. The body started contracting. My mind was full of thoughts and pictures of a rape that happened when I was two and a relative on my mother's side tore my vagina..."*

Thus, the midwifery care or the midwife's attitude, demeanour and responses are extremely important during childbirth. The body of a sexually abused woman has already been violated and tortured once. As a result, she may experience the midwife's care as additional torture and violation. Additionally, phrases spoken by the midwife, e.g., "relax", "nothing to worry about, I'll just feel around a bit to see what the situation is", "it will soon be over, hold on a bit longer" etc., are likely to awaken the subconscious organ memory of the same or similar words being spoken by the perpetrator, under different circumstances – during the sexual abuse [45]. This is why it is highly important that the midwife knows how to ensure safety and that she follows the reactions of the pregnant woman. The midwife needs to be open and accessible for a possible conversation in which she can reassure the mother-to-be that no abuse is taking place and that everything is normal. Above all, she must be respectful. In such moments, it is even better to have someone beside the pregnant woman who knows of her abuse and whom she fully trusts. This person can reassure her that what she is experiencing are reawakened feelings pertaining to her abuse; that the abuse is no longer happening and that it is safe. This double recognition and distinction between the past and the present is extremely important for the mother-to-be [46, 29, 47]. "Flashbacks" can be triggered and reawakened by a touch, words, the position of the woman or the care professional at the maternity hospital or a gynaecological clinic. The woman can react in various ways. She can freeze, become rigid, apathetic, her breathing or facial expressions can change and she can even exhibit signs of panic.

Women who are aware of their abuse and are consciously prepared for these feelings will be able to more easily control the situation. Furthermore, such women will be able to discern that their feelings do not originate in the here and now, but have only been reawakened - it is safe [29, 48].

"My first childbirth was a real nightmare because I couldn't cope with what I was feeling and with my body that failed me completely. When I should have pushed out my baby, I failed, despite numerous attempts, and so the child was born with a CS. When I got pregnant the second time, the push-out was what I was afraid of most. I feared that the same psychical and physical pain would repeat. I started going to therapy and I was set at ease when my therapist helped me understand what transpired during my first childbirth. The pain I felt in my vagina subconsciously reminded me of the pains I felt when, after practice, my coach would grope me and shove in my vagina everything - from his fingers and various objects to his penis. I always considered that part of my body the most dirty and disgusting. When I should have pushed my little baby girl through that space, I was repulsed and couldn't do it, even though time was running out. As long as she was in my belly, she was still pure but then I had the feeling that she would have to swallow all the sperm and all the disgust the coach had given me. With this awareness and strongly determined that my body was clean, while the perpetrator was dirty, I went to give birth for the second time; this time, my son. I gave myself strength with words that my body could not be dirty, ugly and damaged if it was going to give birth to a new life. The birth itself would finally heal old wounds and give me back my dignity as a woman. Although my brain knew all this, the moment the midwife announced that I was fully dilated and ready for the push-out, I started feeling the same horror and anxiety as the first time. As if an invisible force wanted to drag me away again to the world of abuse. I couldn't believe my body would fail me again. I started calling to God for help. And he actually answered. In my mind, I heard the words of my therapist calmly and tenderly resounding: "You are safe now. The earthquake is over. This is only a reawakening of the feelings you were not allowed to feel during abuse...Your uterus is a place where life is born and your body has a remarkable power," she said. "Bring it back into a place of power and life-giving..." And that's how I managed! Prouder than ever in my life, I heard the cry of my second-born child!"

It is much more difficult when a woman is not aware of her abuse. This is because the psyche and body experience are precisely what the woman has suppressed and unprocessed (fear, shame, anxiety, panic, despair, disgust powerlessness, anger, etc.). Clinical practices have shown that many victims of sexual abuse freeze during the abuse itself (a subconscious defence mechanism that helps them survive the difficult events). This is why many victims feel that experiencing the consequences (e.g., flashbacks during pregnancy, childbirth, etc.) is even more traumatic than the original trauma (the abuse). In situations that are subconsciously reminiscent of their past experiences, the flashbacks awaken what they were not allowed to feel during the abuse itself due to apathy and dissociation. This often happens to victims who experience severe pain during their abuse. Consequently, such women may experience dissociation during childbirth. Here, their minds may wonder and they may not feel the pain. They are subconsciously fighting the pain. This can prolong and hinder the course of childbirth. In moments like these, it is very important that the woman can be "present" during childbirth. To do this, her midwife or partner (if he is beside her) need to "calls her back" with words, calm her, tell her she is safe and to believe that all will be fine with her body [45, 29, 47].

"Until the strongest labour pains started intensifying, I was really proud of how well I was doing because I was very afraid of giving birth. But the more the pain grew, the less present I was emotionally. I

suddenly felt I had tuned out into another world even though I didn't want to, but it was as if I had no power or influence any more. Only now and then I still managed to look around and the only thing I remember is the doctor coming to me and calling me by my name. When I heard my name, it seemed as if my brain had realized that I was safe but the body would not obey me. As if it had detached from me. The doctor suggested epidural analgesia and, even though my birth plan said I didn't want it, at that moment, I clung to every kind of help. Truly, the epidural helped me come back and also be emotionally present when my son was born. Having the possibility to decide at the most crucial moment has been one of the most powerful and most positive experiences in my life so far."

Women in therapy often say that, when dissociation occurs, what helps them the most is someone calling them by their name. In the above described case, the epidural analgesia helped because the physical pain (the labour pain), which was reminiscent of the pains during her abuse, triggered dissociation. In other cases, the epidural may cause dissociation or a panic attack. This is because the pregnant woman may feel that she is not in control of her body or that she is, in a way, tied, captured and cannot escape. As a result, she may experience feelings similar to those she experienced during the sexual abuse when her body froze.

Dissociation is strongly associated with the feeling of not being safe: *"I felt as if I followed the entire delivery from outside my body, looking down from the ceiling to the bed where I lay. This made me feel safer. But when contracting and dilating began, I started pushing and crying out for my mother...In my mind, I tried to escape to a safe place...I know it sounds weird, but I couldn't manage being present. I was exhausted from the touches..."*

Physical sensations, such as the stretching of the pelvis, tensions in the body, etc., can strongly remind a woman of, and reawaken, the sexual abuse recorded in her somatic memory – in her body. This impact is stronger and greater if the abuse she suffered involved painful penetrations or rape. General anaesthesia, especially the feeling of losing control over her body, can also arouse fear in a woman with a history of sexual abuse. However, in some cases, general anaesthesia facilitates a woman's ability to cope with childbirth [44].

"My partner and I really looked forward to the childbirth, although we were also afraid about how everything would unfold. I had heard a lot of stories, read a lot of literature, but despite all this I was still completely unprepared for such intense triggers and memories which seemed like a bolt out of the blue. All the horror began when I heard the screaming, bellowing and quick and loud breathing of a woman giving birth in the next room. My chest stung with pain and my heart began pounding with all its force. My legs froze. The more I was supposed to cooperate with the personnel, the more I began to fail. All the old feelings – lying in bed with my legs spread, shouting, panting, pain, the feeling of having no control – and the people around me, whom I was supposed to trust and who were supposed to take care of me, reminded me of the rape I had experienced when I was 12..."

Flashbacks can also be triggered by the **position of the body**, for example lying in bed. A woman who has been sexually abused night after night before sleep, while having to lie on her back in her bed, can experience bad and unpleasant feelings in this position [47].

"The most disgusting thought about giving birth was having to lie naked on my back with my legs apart because, for me, it's the same as rape, with the addition of people walking by and looking into my crotch. The moment I found out who my midwife was going to be, I took a risk and told her what I was most

afraid of and what worried me most. Thank God she was understanding and even thanked me for telling her. Her words that I could give birth also standing up or squatting calmed me so much that there were no more problems or complications because I could relax and believe that it really was safe."

"Until I got into a darkened delivery room, I was fine. But then I suddenly couldn't breathe anymore and the familiar panic and feeling that I'd simply die began intensifying. At that moment, they gave me sedatives so I could cooperate at least somewhat and hear what everyone who came into my room wanted from me. When I was almost completely calm, a bearded older doctor came into the room and my distress began again, but not as intensely. I can't believe that my body failed me again and it seemed as if I was falling into an abyss..."

In therapy, it transcribed that the above mentioned woman had, during her childhood, been sexually abused by her stepfather (man). This man had a beard similar to the doctor and would come into her room in the dark. During her labour, the health professionals entered without knocking or in any other way announcing their entrance, similar to how the perpetrator had come "unannounced".

Most often, the medical personnel is not even aware that they have the power to re-traumatize a woman who has been sexually abused. At the same time, with kindness and professionalism, they can help her experience the delivery as something beautiful. Sometimes a sentence is enough to calm a woman down or, quite the opposite, enough for everything to fall to pieces. Most abused women undergoing therapy report that they find it immensely difficult to tell their midwives or doctors that they have been sexually abused. This is because they are too afraid that the personnel might then look at them funnily or treat them differently. Furthermore, it is likely that some of them have never told anyone about their experience, not even their partner. Many women say that it would be most helpful if, during pregnancy, they had a person (perhaps a doula, a chosen midwife, a determined partner, etc.) who they could communicate their worries and fears to. This person would then be present at delivery. For a mother with a history of sexual abuse, it can be highly reassuring to have someone beside her who knows how she is feeling and understands her reactions to situations which reawaken painful memories. If the mother struggles, this person can speak to the personnel instead of the mother, making the situation "safe" again. When the abuse took place, there was nobody there to protect the girl and provide safety; to speak for her and draw the line or just reassure her that everything would be fine. This is why such a positive experience can be very healing for the victim.

7. Motherhood and the history of sexual abuse

The child is born. Even before giving birth, some mothers are afraid and worry about whether they will be competent mothers, whether they will feel the child, whether they will know how to protect it from dangers, etc. In this section, we explore the studies and clinical experiences relating to sexual abused mothers and their child (during breastfeeding, caring for the child and in their attachment to the child). Furthermore, how they raise their children and how sexual abuse can manifest in subsequent generations.

The first contact after birth is most commonly related to breastfeeding. This involves not only the connection between the mother's and the child's body, but also a very strong emotional bond accompanied by the most varied experiences. If a sexually abused mother feels an aversion to breastfeeding; perhaps this reawakens feelings relating to abuse and reminds her body that someone has been disrespectful to it, then she needs to be given as much support as possible and not be pressured to breastfeed at any cost. Even though her body is completely ready to breastfeed, this does not necessarily mean that her psyche is. This is why emotional contra-indicators need to be taken into account [30].

Accounts of clinical experiences have shown that this often happens to women whose breasts were groped during abuse. As a result, the baby's suckling can act as a trigger that reawakens their fear, anxiety and disgust. Nudity reminds them of how it felt to be exposed and unprotected during abuse. Thus, the first contact between the mother and the child in the maternity hospital, when the baby is laid on the mother's breasts, is extremely important.

"When they laid the child on my breasts immediately after the delivery and tenderly neared its head to the nipple so it began suckling, I felt very comfortable. It meant a lot that the midwife was nice and didn't do anything by force. But the second day in the ward, it was completely different: an unkind nurse grabbed my breast with one hand and the baby's head with the other and pressed the baby on my breast so roughly that it only chocked, while I cried and couldn't say anything, I just froze. In addition, she said that breastfeeding was no science since every animal knew how to feed its young. I was furious with myself for not being able to say anything back to her but I felt so helpless and vulnerable that I cried long after this incident, blaming myself for being a worthless mother who can't protect her newborn child."

Some mothers feel that their milk is dirty because it comes out of their breasts (that were "dirtied" by the perpetrator during abuse). Many mothers feel more relaxed if they have had a daughter, as opposed to a son (because a man abused them and now a "man" is suckling). Other mothers still limit the breastfeeding to daytime. At night they only bottle-feed the baby with pumped milk.

"Strange, but true, I couldn't feed my baby at night because I would find it hard to breathe and I saw in the baby someone who wanted to hurt me. I organically couldn't press it to my bosom. During the day, I didn't experience these feelings at all and I felt like a horrible mother, guilty for having such feelings towards someone completely innocent. Even if I turned on the lights, moved from the bedroom to the living room, it didn't help. Only when I became aware that this was related to my being abused at night; when my father would come to sleep with me because my mother worked the night shift, did the guilt lessen a bit. As long as I breastfed, I was not calm as a mother. I felt much better when the child gradually began eating solid foods and didn't wake up as often during the night."

Clinical experiences show that a similar or an even greater distress is caused by an abused woman's partner's jealousy of their child. This happens during breastfeeding in particular. During breastfeeding, the mother tenderly gives the baby all of her attention. With this, the mother establishes contact through feeding and changing her child, putting it to sleep and cuddling it. A partner who is jealous of this most likely demands attention, exclusively for himself. He may oppress the mother, even when she wants to get up in the middle of the night to comfort and calm the crying baby. He may stand in front of the door, for example, or not allow her to go so as not to "spoil" the child. Even worse, he may demand that she be sexually available to him, perhaps even before her check-up six weeks after the birth and before she is psychically ready.

Women in abusive relationships much more often have an unplanned pregnancy a few months after the birth [49]. Many other studies [18, 50, 51, 44] report that CSA survivors are less content in intimate partner relationships. Overall, there is more discord and violence. Furthermore, there is a higher probability of divorce.

In such a distressful situation, if the mother is lonely and has nobody to support her, she can lose her milk. Furthermore, in order to have some peace from her partner or her awakened feelings, she may decide not to breastfeed anymore. It is extremely important that her environment and medical personnel (the visiting nurse, paediatrician, gynaecologist, etc.) do not judge such a mother or guilt-trip her as this could be devastating for her. This reaction to breastfeeding does not make her a bad mother. If she were to breastfeed, the extreme anxiety she would experience would harm her relationship with her child - far more than not breastfeeding.

"If only I had at the time one person to tell me that I wasn't to blame and that I was a good mother, for I did my best, but I just couldn't manage. Due to the violence I was subjected to daily by my partner and due to his jealous outbursts if I cuddled our child, I stopped breastfeeding because I had constant problems. My baby girl cried because she waited for me to press her to my bosom, but I had to "calm" him first to gain the "right" to breastfeed the child. I was so relieved when he went to work. When the same thing repeated with the second child, I couldn't manage anymore and I got help. I feel better today when he's not here because he went elsewhere. I prefer not to remember that difficult period."

Heightened sensitivity, hormonal changes, sleepless nights, possible discords in the partner relationship, adaptation to the rhythm of feeding and putting the baby to sleep, crying and comforting – any of these strongly affect a mother's wellbeing. However, if the mother has an experience of sexual abuse, it is even harder for her to trust her body and intuition. If she experienced her body already failing her during childbirth, she is even more afraid to trust herself afterwards. She is not sure that she is right about what the child needs when it cries, cannot sleep or refuses to breastfeed. This is precisely why feelings of shame, guilt and anxiety frequently manifest in a sexually abused mother.

All of these feelings are even more present if the woman grew up in a family living in utter chaos or in which everything was wrong and there was no safety. If this was the case, she may develop an intense need to do everything right as a mother. Endeavouring to raise her child differently can lead to extremes – to perfectionism. This can manifest in selfless devotion, that is, in her putting all the child's needs above her own, while suppressing a lot of anger and frustration deep inside her. Such a mother will probably be very critical of how other parents raise their children. She will see herself as different, often stigmatized (as a little girl, she already felt different and stigmatized due to abuse) [49].

The results of a study [52] that measured the parenting characteristics of female survivors of childhood sexual abuse have highlighted some prominent traits: difficulties in setting clear generational boundaries between parents and children, two extreme parenting styles – either permissive parenting or the use of harsh physical discipline. Mothers with a permissive parenting style may avoid invoking parental authority because of their own negative experiences as victims of adult power [53]. They may feel less efficient and "in control" in the parental role. Consequently, they have less confidence in setting appropriate boundaries [54]. Moreover, because they are emotionally more wounded due to the sexual abuse, they have less energy to enforce discipline or appropriate behaviour of their children. They can be easily manipulated by crying children, presumably due to an over-identification with their children's unhappiness [55].

Contrary to this, using physical violence and other harsh parenting methods are likely indicate that the parent is repeating what they were subject to as children. In this, they must not feel the child's pain, for this would mean that they would first have to face the pain they had experienced with their parents. Thus, they subconsciously preserve contact with their parents, albeit in a negative sense, and transmit the patterns of violence [46]. Zuravin et al. [56] suggest something similar. They claim that the maternal history of sexual abuse involving intercourse is related to the increased chances of physical abuse, sexual abuse or neglect in the second generation.

"I remember my aunt telling me once that my mother had been raped as a teenager. I can't understand how this experience didn't make her protect me from the abuses of my father and brother. As if she didn't know what it meant for someone to dirty you like that and seal your fate?! Once, when she came into my room, she saw what my father was doing to me, but she just closed the door, went away and never said anything. THIS hurt me even more than everything I experienced from my father and brother. And I felt guilty, as if I was stealing her husband. I feel sick just thinking about it. She was so cruel as a mother. I fear whether I'll know how to protect my daughter so that nothing like that ever happens to her."

Additionally, children of abused mothers are often parental, taking care of the emotional needs of their mothers who are, in a way, emotionally dependent on them (no healthy boundaries). Compared to their peers, these children look much more grown up. However, in the long term, their own development can suffer [57]. Clinical experiences show that mothers often treat their children as confidants and friends. This is particularly the case if they do not get along with their partner. Mothers reporting a history of incest were more likely to interact with their sons in a subtly seductive manner, considered to be indicative of generational boundary dissolution [58].

"Until recently, my mother and I were best friends. She confided everything in me, even the sexual problems they had with my father. How I felt or what went on with me never interested her. She often even said that if she hadn't had me, she'd have rather died. She was jealous of my friends who were never good enough for me. I thought all this was normal, even more, it seemed a special privilege that not all daughters were entitled to. But when I was treated for bulimia, I discovered what she did to me. She attended the sessions a few times and the therapist discovered that just like she overstepped all emotional limits with me, so a man in her childhood overstepped all limits with her, also in the sexual sense."

In general, children of sexually abused mothers show a more helpful, protective, managing and controlling behaviours towards family members. On the other hand, children of non-abused mothers show significantly more trusting, deferring, relying and submitting behaviours [59]. Grocke, Smith and Graham [60] have found that, compared to children of non-abused mothers, children of CSA survivors are more prone to interpreting ambiguous pictures of children and strangers as negative or frightening. They also believe that sexually abused mothers teach their children about the male and female sexual development and contraception-related topics in more detail. Such mothers find this increased communication essential. This is because they presume that it will protect their children from a experiencing a similar sexual abuse. On the contrary, Douglas [61] reports that mothers with a history of sexual abuse are more anxious in child care, requiring intimate contact such as changing, bathing and putting to bed. Even though these activities, as such, are not "sexual", they may indicate that, because of the mother's unease, sexuality and intimacy will be taboo topics in the child's growing up.

Women who are aware of having been sexually abused may often fear that they will themselves **abuse** their child. The fact that the mother is afraid is a sort of safeguard and it is, therefore, quite unlikely that she would sexually abuse her child. However, there can be situations in which she feels aroused. For example, during the changing, bathing or breastfeeding of her child. Her body tells her that what is happening is not natural, that it is perverted. Particularly, this can happen if she, herself, has been sexually abused on the changing table. In this case, she may not even have the images in her explicit memory, that is, she cannot recall the event of the abuse. It suffices that her body remembers it, that the abuse is recorded in the organ memory - in implicit memory. If arousal or disgust occur, it is important that the mother controls herself, that she takes time to evaluate her feelings. In other words, it is necessary that she sets boundaries and becomes aware that it is her abuse reawakening; that her child deserves pure love. She has to feel able to withdraw, go to her partner and communicate these feelings if she is unable to process them herself. When this does not work, it is necessary that the mother seeks the help of a professional who will assist her in going through the emotions of abuse (disgust, shame, etc.) and help her work through them. It is not necessary for inappropriate touching to occur during the changing or bathing of the child, the atmosphere can already become terrifying and abusive when the mother feels aroused by the child's innocent and powerless body (just like someone who sexually abused her as a little girl was aroused by her as an innocent and powerless child). At the same time, the mother feels contempt for and disgust with herself for having these feelings. These feelings and real bodily sensations are unfair, both on the mother who experiences them and on the child who, through the projection-introjection identification, senses and feels her distress or, even more, when the child drinks these feelings of abuse on her bosom [29]. In such an atmosphere, it is more likely that the unresolved feelings (perhaps even the action itself) will lead to an intergenerational transmission of the trauma of sexual abuse, which we will discuss in the next section.

8. Intergenerational transmission of the trauma of sexual abuse and motherhood

Johnson [62] claims that people who are victims of emotional, physical or sexual abuse are six times more likely to continue the abuse they have suffered. Other studies [63] have shown that half of the mothers whose children have been sexually abused have, themselves, been victims of sexual abuse. If the act of sexual abuse is not transmitted, this does not mean that the children of sexually abused parents will be safe from sexual abusers. Relational family therapy [16] discusses the unresolved effects of abuse, including disgust, shame and anger. These are vertically transmitted from the abused parent to the child through the mechanism of projection-introjection identification. Even if this parent tries to warn the child about all the dangers of abuse [64], but is not in touch with the unprocessed effects and therefore does not know how to protect him/herself and set boundaries, it is much more likely that the child will become a victim of sexual abuse [16]. Miller suggests something similar in her *The Body Never Lies: The Lingering Effects of Hurtful Parenting* [65]. Here, she argues that childhood abuse is resolved in two ways: grown-ups who have been sexually abused as children transmit their unacknowledged emotions to their children or other people around them. Alternatively, the effects are suffered by the body of the abused person with psychosomatic or chronic diseases. In his study, Cross [55] reports that 34% of mothers whose children have been sexually abused have, themselves, been victims of sexual abuse. In their work, McCloskey and Bailey [66], state that it is three to four times more likely that a daughter of a mother who was a victim of sexual abuse would herself would be sexually abused, than in cases when mothers had no experience of sexual abuse. They believe that a common reason for the transmission of sexual abuse between generations is the preservation and continuation of contacts with the family members involved in the sexual abuse of the mother and then, also, the daughter. Other studies have shown that mothers of children who had been sexually abused like them exhibit a higher degree of stress and symptoms of post-traumatic stress disorder [67]. Additionally, they express fear that they will be bad mothers, directing hostility and frustrations towards their children [55]. Sexually abused mothers also show difficulties establishing a structure, expressing affection and love for their children. They feel mixed emotions towards them and fear that their children will also become victims. This often results in them socially isolating their children, in order to protect them [55]. The results of a study by Hall, Sachs and Rayens [68] show that mothers with a history of sexual abuse use physical punishment on their children six times more often than mothers who have not been sexually abused. Cohen [69] stresses that, if they have not worked through the abuse, sexually abused mothers are less skilful and functional in the parental role.

One of the responses to an unprocessed sexual abuse can also be seen in the mother's negative behaviour towards the child. For example, if the mother has been sexually abused as a little girl just as she started saying her first words, she may subconsciously feel an intense dislike and negative attitude towards her child when it starts to talk. She will not know what is going on but her body will testify to her distress. If she is able to take this distress seriously and allow herself to feel the girl inside her, then she will be able to accept her child. If not, this rejection and refusal of the child may intensify to a degree of neglect [30].

Some cases of unprocessed and repressed sexual abuse of a mother can come to light when, at a certain age, a child begins to frequently get ill or when various psychosomatic signs appear, sometimes also behavioural or learning problems. Usually the age at which certain symptoms emerge, (e.g., headaches, bedwetting, troubles sleeping etc.) coincides with the age at which the mother was sexually abused. With an ailing child, the mother may feel powerlessness, fear and even anger for having to keep going to the doctors. However, all of these feelings actually belong to her sexual abuse. Her child merely activates and reawakens them as they have not yet been processed. This is because she is not in contact with them. As a girl, when her body was exposed and unprotected, she felt fear and powerlessness. She had to suppress her anger at an injustice she suffered. When she senses the child's distress and sympathizes with it, she will help herself and contribute to the resolution of the feelings from her abuse. This will help not only her child, but also the little girl still living inside her who never really received any compassion, safety and support.

9. Conclusion

The body never forgets sexual abuse. Even if the psyche pushes it to the subconscious because the pain is too great, the body will cry for help in every possible way (through psychosomatic troubles, health issues, addiction, workaholism, conflicts in a partner relationship, depressions, etc.). Years, even decades, can go by before the consequences of the abuse surface. If the abused woman functions normally, it may seem that she has no problems. However, one trigger, like pregnancy or childbirth, may suffice for sensations and feelings similar to the ones during the sexual abuse to start uncontrollably emerging. Most survivors do not even relate this to the original trauma, looking for the causes somewhere else completely. Yet, the problem is not solved until the trauma is. In the safe and trusting therapeutic environment, there is a way out of the vicious circle of distress and pain. However, it is a long process for which the abused needs a lot of strength, determination, resolution and encouragement, especially when the occasional crises occur. Clinical experiences have shown that, with an in-depth and successful therapy, an individual can live a very good and decent life. After successful therapy, they feel that they finally have "control" over the past - and not the other way round. At the same time, due to the distinction between the present (when something merely awakens) and the past (when something actually happened), such a person is much more relaxed as a parent. She can trust her intuition and body and feel her child as a mother. This means, of course, that she does everything to protect the child from experiencing a violence similar to the one she had. She emotionally equips the child so it is able to go out into the world. She ensures to sever the intergenerational transmission of the trauma of sexual abuse.

Author details

Tanja Repič Slavič* and Christian Gostečnik

*Address all correspondence to: tanjarepic@gmail.com

Chair of Marital and Family Therapy, Department of Psychology and Sociology of Religion, Faculty of Theology, University of Ljubljana, Slovenia

References

[1] Williams LM. 'Recall of Childhood Trauma: A Prospective Study of Women's Memories of Child Sexual Abuse.' *Journal of Consulting and Clinical Psychology* 1994:62(6) 1167-76.

[2] *Združenje Proti Spolnemu Zlorabljanju. Spolna Zloraba Otrok.* http://www.spolnonasilje.over.net/zgibanke/spolnost.htm. 2007. (accessed January 23 2007).

[3] Adams-Tucker C. 'A Socioclinical Overview of 28 Sex-abused Children.' *Child Abuse and Neglect* 1981:5 361-7.

[4] Browne A, Finkelhor D. 'Initial and Long-term Effects: A Review of the Research.' In: David Finkelhor, ed. *A Sourcebook on Child Sexual Abuse.* Beverly Hills: CA: Sage; 1986.

[5] Conte JR, Schuerman JR. 'Factors Associated with an Increased Impact of Child Sexual Abuse.' *Child Abuse & Neglect* 1987:11(2) 201-11.

[6] Pierce R, Pierce LH. 'The Sexually Abused Child: A Comparison of Male and Female Victims.' *Child Abuse & Neglect* 1985:9(2) 191-9.

[7] Bass E, Davis L. *Pogum za Okrevanje: Priro nik za ženske, ki so Preživele Spolno Zlorabo v Otroštvu (The Courage to Heal: A Guide for Women Survivors of Child Sexual Abuse.)* Prev. Polona Mesec. Ljubljana: Liberalna Akademija, Visoka šola za Socialno Delo; 1998.

[8] Catherall DR. *Handbook of Stress, Trauma, and the Family.* New York: Brunner-Routledge; 2004.

[9] Corby B. *Child Abuse Towards a Knowledge Base*. Buckingham: Open University Press; 2006.

[10] Courtois CA. *Healing the Incest Wound: Adult Survivors in Therapy.* New York: W. W. Norton & Company; 1996.

[11] Scaer R. *The Trauma Spectrum: Hidden Wounds and Human Resiliency.* New York, NY: W. W. Norton & Company; 2005.

[12] Schore AN. 'Early Relational Trauma, Disorganized Attachment, and the Development of a Predisposition to Violence'. In: Daniel J. Siegel and Marion F. Solomon, ed. Healing *Trauma: Attachment, Mind, Body, and Brain,* 107-67. New York: W. W. Norton & Company; 2003.

[13] Van der Kolk BA. 'The Body Keeps the Score: Memory and the Evolving Psychobiology of Post Traumatic Stress.' *Harvard Review of Psychiatry* 1994:1(5) 253-65.

[14] Rodgers CS, Lang AJ, Twamley EW, Stein MB. 'Sexual Trauma and Pregnancy: A Conceptual Framework.' *Journal of Women's Health* 2003:12(10) 961-70.

[15] Golding JM. 'Sexual Assault History and Physical Health in Randomly Selected Los Angeles Women.' *Health Psychology* 1994:13(2) 130-8.

[16] Goste nik C. *Relacijska Družinska Terapija (Relational Family Therapy).* Ljubljana: Brat Fran išek in Fran iškanski Družinski Inštitut; 2004.

[17] Brener ND, McMahon PM, Warren CW, Douglas KA. 'Forced Sexual Intercourse and Associated Health-risk Behaviors Among Female College Students in the United States.' *Journal of Consulting and Clinical Psychology* 1999:67(2) 252-9.

[18] Briere J, Evans D, Runtz M, Wall T. 'Symptomatology in Men who were Molested as Children: A Comparison Study.' *American Journal of Orthopsychiatry* 1988:58(3) 457-61.

[19] Noll JG, Trickett PK, Putnam FW. 'A Prospective Investigation of the Impact of Childhood Sexual Abuse on the Development of Sexuality.' *Journal of Consulting and Clinical Psychology* 2003:71 575-86.

[20] Saewyc EM, Magee LL, Pettingall SE. 'Teenage Pregnancy and Associated Risk Behavior Among Sexually Abused Adolescents.' *Perspectives on Sexual and Reproductive Health* 2004: 36(3) 98-105.

[21] Stock JL, Bell MA, Boyer DK, Connell FA. 'Adolescent Pregnancy and Sexual Risk-Taking Among Sexually Abused Girls.' *Family Planning Perspectives* 1997:29(5) 200-3.

[22] Seng JS, Oakley DJ, Sampselle CM, Killion C, Graham-Bermann S, Liberzon I. Posttraumatic stress disorder and pregnancy complications. Obstetrics & Gynecology 2001:97(1) 17-22.

[23] Möhler E, Matheis V, Marysko M, Finke P, Kaufmann C, Cierpka M, Reck C, Resch F. 'Complications During Pregnancy, Peri- and Postnatal Period in a Sample of Women with a History of Child Abuse.' J*ournal of Psychosomatic Obstetrics Gynaecology* 2008:29(3) 193-8.

[24] Grimstad H, Schei B. 'Pregnancy and Delivery for Women with a History of Child Sexual Abuse.' *Child Abuse Neglect* 1999:23(1) 81-90.

[25] Spinelli MG. 'Interpersonal Psychotherapy for Depressed Antepartum Women: A Pilot Study.' *American Journal of Psychiatry* 1997:154(7) 1028-30.

[26] Goldschmidt L, Day NL, Richardson GA. 'Effects of Prenatal Marijuana Exposure on Child Behavior Problems at Age 10.' *Neurotoxicology and Teratology* 2000:22(3) 25-36.

[27] Waugh E, Bulik CM. 'Offspring of Women with Eating Disorders.' *International Journal of Eating Disorders* 1999:25(2) 123-33.

[28] Neff K. PTSD: 'Survivors of Sexual Abuse and Pregnancy.' 2010. http://www.examiner.com/article/ptsd-survivors-of-sexual-abuse-and-pregnancy (accessed June 15 2014).

[29] Repi T. *Nemi Kriki Spolne Zlorabe in Novo Upanje (The Silent Cry of Sexual Abuse and a New Hope*). Založba Mohorjeva Družba: Celje; 2008.

[30] Prescott A. 'Childhood Sexual Abuse and the Potential Impact on Maternity.' *Midwifery Matters* 2002:92 17-9.

[31] Wijma K, Wijma B, Zar M. 'Psychometric Aspects of the W-DEQ; A New Questionnaire for the Measurement of Fear of Childbirth.' *Journal of Psychosomatic Obstetrics & Gynecology* 1998:19(2) 84-97.

[32] Heimstad R, Dahloe R, Laache I, Skogvoll E, Schei B. 'Fear of Childbirth and History of Abuse: Implications for Pregnancy and Delivery.' *Acta Obstetricia et Gynecologica Scandinavica* 2006:85(4) 435-40.

[33] Areskog B, Uddenberg N, Kjessler B. 'Background Factors in Pregnant Women With and Without Fear of Childbirth.' *Journal of Psychosomatic Obstetrics & Gynecology* 1983:2(2) 102-108.

[34] Melender HL. 'Experiences of Fears Associated with Pregnancy and Childbirth: A Study of 329 Pregnant Women.' *Birth* 2002:29(2) 101-111.

[35] Lukasse M, Vangen S, Øian P, Kumle M, Ryding EL, Schei B. 'Childhood Abuse and Fear of Childbirth--a Population-based Study.' *Birth* 2010:37(4) 267-274.

[36] Leeners B, Richter-Appelt H, Imthurn B, Rath W. 'Influence of Childhood Sexual Abuse on Pregnancy, Delivery, and the Early Postpartum Period in Adult Women.' *Journal of Psychosomatic Research* 2006:61(2) 139-51.

[37] Jacobs JL. 'Child Sexual Abuse Victimization and Later Sequelae During Pregnancy and Childbirth.' *Journal of Child Sexual Abuse* 1992:1(1) 103-12.

[38] Rhodes N, Hutchinson S. 'Labor Experiences of Childhood Sexual Abuse Survivors.' *Birth* 1994:21(4) 213-20.

[39] Tallman N, Hering C. Child Abuse and Its Effects on Birth. New Research. Midwifery Today Int Midwife 1998:45 19-21.

[40] Saisto T, Kaaja R, Ylikorkala O, Halmesmaki E. 'Reduced Pain Tolerance During and After Pregnancy in Women Suffering from Fear of Labor.' *Pain* 2001:93(2) 123-7.

[41] Zar M, Wijma K, Wijma B. 'Pre- and Postpartum Fear of Childbirth in Nulliparous and Parous women.' *Scandinavian Journal of Behavioral Therapy* 2001:30(2) 75-84.

[42] Laursen M, Johansen C, Hedegaard M. 'Fear of Childbirth and Risk for Birth Complications in Nulliparous Women in the Danish National Birth Cohort.' *BJOG: An International Journal of Obstetrics and Gynaecology* 2009:116(10) 1350-1355.

[43] Soet JE, Brack GA, Dilorio C. 'Prevalence and Predictors of Women's Experience of Psychological Trauma During Childbirth.' *Birth* 2003:30(1) 36-46.

[44] Smith M. 'Childbirth in Women with a History of Sexual Abuse (I).' *Practising Midwife* 1998:1(5) 20-3.

[45] Courtois CA, Courtois-Riley C. 'Pregnancy and Childbirth as Triggers for Abuse Memories: Implications for Care.' *Birth* 1992:19(4) 222-3.

[46] Goste nik C. *Relacijska Paradigma in Travma (Relational Paradigm and Trauma).* Ljubljana: Brat Fran išek in Fran iškanski Družinski Inštitut; 2009.

[47] Tilley J. 'Sexual Assault and Flashbacks on the Labour Ward.' *Practising Midwife* 2000:3(4) 18-20.

[48] Repi Slavi T, Goste nik C, Cvetek R. 'Trauma of Sexual abuse and the Family.' In: SPITERI, Ylenia (ed.), GALEA, Elizabeth M. (ed.). *Psychology of Neglect, (Psychology Research Progress).* New York: Nova Science, cop.; 2012. p.29-46, Available from https://www.novapublishers.com/catalog/product_info.php?products_id=28684. (accessed December 2 2012).

[49] Washington Coalition of Sexual Assault Programs (WCSAP). *Pregnant and Parenting Survivors.* http://www.wcsap.org/pregnant-and-parenting-survivors. 2014 (accessed June 16 2014).

[50] DiLillo D, Long PJ. 'Perceptions of Couple Functioning Among Female Survivors of Child Sexual Abuse.' *Journal of Child Sexual Abuse* 1999:7 59-76.

[51] Finkelhor D, Hotaling GT, Lewis IA, Smith C. 'Sexual Abuse in a National Survey of Adult Men and Women: Prevalence, Characteristics and Risk factors.' *Child Abuse & Neglect* 1990:14 19-28.

[52] DiLillo D, Damashek A. *Parenting Characteristics of Women Reporting a History of Childhood Sexual Abuse.* University of Nebraska – Lincoln. Faculty Publications, Department of Psychology. http://digitalcommons.unl.edu/cgi/viewcontent.cgi?article=1106&context=psychfacpub: 2003 (accessed June 15 2014).

[53] Ruscio AM. 'Predicting the Child-rearing Practices of Mothers Sexually Abused in Childhood.' *Child Abuse & Neglect* 2001:25 369-387.

[54] Cole PM, Woolger C, Power TG, Smith KD. 'Parenting Difficulties Among Incest Survivors of Father-daughter Incest.' *Child Abuse & Neglect* 1992:16 239-49.

[55] Cross W. 'A Personal History of Childhood Sexual Abuse: Parenting Patterns and Problems.' *Clinical Child Psychology and Psychiatry* 2001:6(4) 563-74.

[56] Zuravin S, McMillen C, DePanfilis D, Risley-Curtiss C. 'The Intergenerational Cycle of Maltreatment: Continuity Versus Discontinuity.' *Journal of Interpersonal Violence* 1996:11 315-334.

[57] Chase ND. *Burdened Children: Theory, Research, and Treatment of Parentification.* Thousand Oaks, CA: Sage;1999.

[58] Sroufe LA, Jacobvitz D, Mangelsdorf S, De Angelo E, Ward MJ. 'Generational Boundary Dissolution Between Mothers and their Preschool Children: A Relationship Systems Approach.' *Child Development* 1985:56 317-325.

[59] Burkett LP. 'Parenting Behaviors of Women Who Were Sexually Abused as Children in Their Families of Origin.' *Journal of Family Process* 1991:30(4) 421-34.

[60] Grocke M, Smith M, Graham P. 'Sexually Abused and Nonabused Mother's Discussions about Sex and their Children's Sexual Knowledge.' *Child Abuse & Neglect* 1995:19 985-996.

[61] Douglas AR. 'Reported Anxieties Concerning Intimate Parenting in Women Sexually Abused as Children.' *Child Abuse & Neglect* 2000:24 425-34.

[62] Johnson TC. 'Some Considerations About Sexual Abuse and Children with Sexual Behavior Problems.' In: James A. Chu and Elizabeth S. Bowman, ed. *Trauma and Sexuality: The Effects of Childhood Sexual, Physical, and Emotional Abuse on Sexual Identity and Behavior*, 83-106. New York: The Haworth Medical Press; 2002.

[63] Collin-Vezina D. 'Current Understanding about Intergenerational Transmission of Child Sexual Abuse.' *Child Abuse and Neglect* 2003:27(5) 489-508.

[64] Howell EF. '»Good Girls,« Sexy »Bad Girls,« and Warriors: The Role of Trauma and Dissociation in the Creation and Reproduction of Gender.' In: James A. Chu and Elizabeth S. Bowman, ed. *Trauma and Sexuality: The Effects of Childhood Sexual, Physical, and Emotional Abuse on Sexual Identity and Behavior*, 5-32. New York: The Haworth Medical Press;2002.

[65] Miller A. *Upor telesa: Telo terja resnico (The Body Never Lies: The Lingering Effects of Hurtful Parenting).* Prev. Rapa Šuklje. Ljubljana: Tangram;tra2005.

[66] McCloskey LA, Bailey JA. 'The Intergenerational Transmission of Risk for Child Sexual Abuse.' *Journal of Interpersonal Violence* 2000:15(10) 1019-35.

[67] Timmons-Mitchell J, Chandler-Holtz D, Semple WE. 'Post-traumatic Stress Symptoms in Mothers Following Children's Reports of Sexual Abuse: An Exploratory Study.' *American Journal of Orthopsychiatry* 1996:66(3) 463-7.

[68] Hall LA, Sachs B, Rayens MK. 'Mothers' Potential for Child Abuse: The Roles of Childhood Abuse and Social Resources.' *Nursing Research* 1998:47(2) 87-95.

[69] Cohen M, Deamant C, Barkan S, Richardson J, Young M, Holman S, Anastos K, Cohen J, Melnick S. 'Domestic Violence and Childhood Sexual Abuse in HIV-infected Women and Women at Risk for HIV.' American Journal of Public Health 2000:90(4) 560-5.

Chapter 7

Female Sexuality and Medicine – Sexualisation of Everyday Life, Desexualisation of Childbirth

Zalka Drglin

Additional information is available at the end of the chapter

http://dx.doi.org/10.5772/60124

1. Introduction

There is a widespread belief that doctors are the "real" experts on women's health, sexual health included, and that biomedicine holds the key to improving it. This paper is going to demonstrate the limitations of such an approach, challenging the common perception that medicine alone holds the key to understanding women's sexuality. In considering women's sexuality we have to step outside the biomedical model to explore the ways in which some theories and practices are silenced and others are (re)produced.

The paper will seek answers to the fundamental question about the bond between women and medicine from the perspective of the everyday life of the modern woman: What does medicine have to do with female liberation, particularly in the field of sexuality? We are dealing with complex questions; it is a challenging task to maintain the tension of the controversies and avoid over-simplification. We are particularly interested in the idea of the regulation of female sexuality, and hence the patriarchal management of female bodies through the State and its institutions. This paper will elaborate the idea that one important part of modernization is the regulation, management and surveillance of the human body, with sexuality a particularly prominent feature. Medicine plays an important role in those processes. We are going to explore our topic from multiple points of view, historical, sociological and cultural, with use of concepts like sex/gender, knowledge, power, embodiment, and medicalization. Female sexuality and its controversial bonds with medicine have to be in the centre of interest for those who are dedicated to women's well-being, especially in times of life transitions such as puberty, childbirth and menopause.

2. The sexualization of everyday life

Let us begin with a short overview of the sexualization of various aspects of everyday life, followed by a look into the controversial links between female sexuality and medicine. Considering the proliferation of sexual messages surrounding us and their use as bait to get consumers to purchase products, whether they are needed or not, it is tempting to see the sex lives of modern individuals as being free from any and all taboos, as if reservations no longer apply – satisfaction and instant gratification are made freely available and cater to every taste, every kind of sexual desire. Sexuality is marketed as a commodity, bought *en masse* and sold on a grand scale.

On the surface, sex and sexual activity are presented as a private matter of individuals and a question of personal choice. The achievements of second-wave feminism [1], along with the accomplishments of the "sexual revolution" (a mass movement of the younger generations in Western Europe and the US between 1964 and 1975, which advocated for "free love", free from traditionalist patterns of sexual behaviour and some of its taboos) have gone down in 20th century history [2] as significant events for women's equality, including in terms of sexuality. For the subject at hand, we can mention specific areas such as violence, including rape [3] (as a form of specific sexualized violence used, among other things, for the reproduction of power relations between genders in the patriarchal family and society), and productive rights (especially safe and reliable birth control, safe abortion and the accessibility thereof to a wide range of women), as well as the questioning of myths about motherhood [4]. This primarily involved the pursuit of the conditions for an active heterosexual life for women, unaffected by unwanted, involuntary motherhood. At the same time, prejudice about socially undesirable or unlawful sexual practices of the time, such as sex before marriage, teenage sexual activity and homosexual love, was being dismantled. The revolutionary undoing of inhibitions in favour of freer sexual expression also meant the undermining of patriarchal sexual attitudes, which signalled a chance for greater autonomy of women, and was supported by the women's health movement in its attempts to establish a body of knowledge different from oppressive medical discourses and practices, including on women's sexuality [5].

Where do we stand now? It seems that we have gone from prohibiting certain aspects of sexuality to imposing sexuality in many aspects of our lives, that sex has been incorporated into the general wave of consumerism and hyper-spending as one form of escapism for the modern individual in today's consumerist society [6]. Modern individuals who are incapable of sufficient self-reflection are exposed to compulsory consumption of all kinds of sexually informed messages, from enormous billboards to short commercial text messages, which use imagery and words to arouse desire solely in order to make consumers spend more and be easier to manipulate. Clever pop mimicry of free, genuine and primal sex, purported to be the essence of free sexuality, has lured in those seeking an escape. They face constant temptation to answer the persistent call to "Choose and enjoy yourself!" based on the nihilist principle of "Everything is permitted" – albeit with the caveat "Only if you have money" in the small print.

What has been proclaimed as liberating has also created new potential for fresh forms of control and subjugation. It is not too much of a stretch to say that the potential of free sexuality to enable and embody social progress has been overstated or, at the very least, skilfully diverted. The accomplishments of the sexual revolution have been exploited by neoliberalism to gain new, previously inconceivable profits on the pornography market for example [7], as well as by the proliferating global sex trade, ranging from prostitution to sex trafficking, which treats particularly vulnerable groups, including children, women, the economically disadvantaged and other individuals whose very existence is under threat, as goods, and ruthlessly subjugates them to the logic of the market. At the same time, new technologies have provided new channels for sexual messages, in particular via the Internet, which advances the spread of compulsory sexuality and aggravates phenomena like sex addiction [8].

3. Is female sexuality now free of any and all taboos and coercion?

We assert that the aforementioned issues do not affect both genders to the same degree; answers need to be provided to questions about how female sexuality and procreation in general should be perceived and experienced, and about the role played by medicine in these issues. Living a fulfilling life often involves the ability to decide how to express one's own sexuality in all its shifts throughout life cycles, and to find opportunities to live out that sexuality in relationships on a personal and interpersonal level. The question is, however, whether our personal, intimate and individual sex lives really exist within the sphere of freedom. Many things we may see as spontaneous are not truly spontaneous – we are born into a certain environment which shapes our idea of female and male sexuality through cultural, social, domestic and religious convictions. Beliefs, moral judgements, preferences all shape a number of key relationships between individuals and culture(s) as a consequence of a variety of complex and interconnected factors permeating families, institutions concerned with education and health, the media and so on. The (self-)perception of individuals and their relationship to their own gender, the gender of others and sexuality are linked to responsibility and respect felt for oneself and other human beings – what I (do not) like about myself and others, what I (do not) appreciate myself and others, what I am worth, what is male and female sexuality, what is sexually (un-)appealing, what a sexually (un-)appealing body looks like, what the relations between pleasure, gratification, passion, a sense of belonging, validation and love are.

Human sexuality cannot be reduced to the mere sex act; it involves more than just genitals and procreation. The history of sexual desire tells us that the desire to experience sexual pleasure and total body sex – that is, the expansion of sexuality from a limited focus on the face and genitals to include the entire body – has been known since antiquity [9] and was, disregarding the period of the repression of sexual desire in Christian Europe, kept alive up to its renaissance in the 19th century, which continues to this day. Sexual activity is also importantly affected by sexual desire, which goes beyond a mere instinct: the sex act, be it heterosexual or homosexual, is never a mere spontaneous, instinct-driven biological act; it is necessarily a socially conditioned, complex act with its own symbolic value [10]. Researchers of sexuality have yet to agree on the question of whether there are any differences in sexual desire between men and women, and if so, whether they are caused by nature or nurture. On a hormonal level, sexual desire is linked to androgens, which are produced in testicles, in men, and androgens and oestrogen in women, produced in ovaries, as well as testosterone and oxytocin. According to some studies, how we experience sexuality may also be gender-specific, but although the belief that men are more sexual than women, and the principal initiators of sex, while women are more passive, and recipients, is still prevalent in some places, it has become increasingly clear that the differences are differences in the expression of sexuality, which is informed by the culture and social (gendered) roles as well as the expected sexual behaviour for men and women. The belief that women's erogenous zones are more widely dispersed on the body than in men is also prevalent. The way women perceive themselves and their own sexuality is also influenced by prevailing culture – women learn to be passive. They respond to visual and other impulses and become aroused as quickly as men, but being sexually liberated is much more socially acceptable for men. Myths persist about female sexuality in relation to the idea that women have a greater need to form an emotional bond.

Where do we currently stand with regard to female sexuality, socially speaking? There are, of course, multiple types of discourse, and we can highlight the abuse of female sexuality on multiple levels, including devaluation, objectification, the focus on the physical female body in the media, and the propagating of a certain ideal female appearance, which currently means a slim body with no cellulite and the right curves in the right places, with shifting ideas of how much curviness is still acceptable. In addition, female sexuality is constantly being redefined, still seen as goods to be traded in order to survive, to provide protection or sometimes to climb the social ladder; in traditionalist environments, female sexuality is the expression of a woman's worth or worthlessness, as evidenced by the revival of the cult of virginity, which must be maintained until entering a monogamous relationship [11]. Even today, the myth of supposedly passive female sexuality as opposed to active male sexuality persists in popular culture; at the same time, female sexuality is perceived as mysterious, or demonized and regarded as a threat to men. Messages in the media reinforce the chosen model of female sexuality through culturally selected behavioural patterns for each gender and selected sexually informed images that only emphasise certain kinds of sexual expression. This model is perpetuated through various types of discourse about the necessity of maintaining health, beauty and youthfulness through self-discipline and through the simultaneous popularization of the post-modern commandment of "Enjoy yourself!"

It is vital to continuously recollect relevant thoughts of feminist authors about the female body, sexuality, health, and motherhood, which take issue with the culturally prevalent "self-evident" and "common-sense" concepts of sex, which are frequently based on the idea of duality and opposition and on the inequality and imbalance of both sides: nature vs. culture, woman vs. man, sex vs. gender. To mention some: Simone de Beauvoir, Adrienne Rich, Shulamith Firestone, Gena Corea, Evelyn Fox Keller, Emily Martin, Ann Oakley, and Barbara Katz Rothman. We must work towards fighting this amnesia, for to forget the findings about the cultural basis of the dominant understanding of sex, bodies and sexuality, which are the result of numerous excursions into these topics in history, sociology, anthropology, cultural studies and the social history of medicine (Edward Shorter), the history of the body (Thomas Laqueur), the history of the family and birth (Phillip Ariès, Jacques Gélis) and the sociology

http://dx.doi.org/10.5772/60124

of the body (Bryan S. Turner) in particular, would be to accept shallow thought and a superficial reflection of everyday life, the breeding grounds for the myths of a passive masochistic female sexual nature, lower sexual needs of women and monogamous femininity, as opposed to the male, biologically dictated polygamy whose representation has seen a recent revival in some popular media, for example.

4. Sexuality and health

Sexuality is also linked to health issues. People have general health needs regardless of gender, but also face limitations on various levels in meeting those needs and providing the optimal conditions to lead a healthy, or, more generally, a comfortable life, including sexuality.

Both genders have specific health needs; however, women's health has an additional dimension to it due to their reproductive capacity. Throughout history, women have often been reduced to their bodies and their specific biological capacity for procreation (S. de Beauvoir). According to Edward Shorter, a professor of social history of medicine, in his famous work *Women's Bodies* [12], women were victims of their own bodies for centuries, adding that pregnancy, labour and gynaecological diseases constituted high risks. Women could not live out their sexuality due to dismal living conditions and the risks posed to their well-being or life, which also provided grounds for the oppression of women by men. Women were more vulnerable and therefore more closely controlled due to their potential or actual motherhood. Both the biological capacity of the female body to procreate and the social implications of this are more pronounced and more closely linked to subjugation than the biological and social role played by men in procreation. An influential French historian focusing on the history of women, motherhood and sexuality, Yvonne Knibiehler, points out that mothers, motherhood and the "production" of children are stakes of those of power [13]. Control over female fertility is an excellent example of the domination of one gender by the other from a privileged position of power.

5. Knowledge and science about women

Hatred or dislike of women has formed the basis for sexist prejudice and ideology serving as justification for the oppression of females in male-dominated societies throughout the long history of our culture; as in the first era of feminism and feminist theory, the reconstruction of knowledge is now at the forefront. The female has been the gender more closely associated with physicality throughout history; that is, the idea of the female is less easily separated from the body than that of the male. This is why it is all the more important to evaluate the investments of science into the reproductive capacity of women, pregnancy, labour and motherhood, as well as female sexuality. In large part this means reconstructing knowledge about the female body in certain scientific fields and expanding our understanding of multiple links between types of discourse and institutional practices which view the female body through the lens of its sexual and procreative functions.

In particular, light needs to be shed on the way our physical "nature" – an indivisible union of biology and nature shaped by human evolution – is shaped, reinforced or repressed by social conditioning. Most of the time, nature and nurture have simultaneous effects, and the filtering and profiling of what can and cannot be expressed also contributes to every culturally specific definition of male and female sexuality. Carefully thinking about the nature of the physical does away with the expectation that removing historical layers from the cultural conceptualization of masculinity and femininity should lead us to the (pre-)historical, pure, natural male and female body [14, 15]. The simplified sex-neutral history of the human body needs to be disregarded [16]. Let us introduce our reflections on female sexuality and medicine by paraphrasing the famed phrase "the body has a history" (of sociology of the body) [17] – "the body has a herstory, too". We have to speak about *historicized* bodies. The body is a location of control and the exercise of both social and medical power; the social and the medical aspects frequently cannot be told apart, because the medical point of view, as regards the modern idea of health and the individualization of responsibility for health and illness, is inherently linked to social control over the health of the population(s) [17, 18].

The history of women is characterized by the desire to exercise control over them and their reproductive functions, in different aspects such as pregnancy, childbirth, and motherhood [19-23]. This means, for example, that the patriarchal social order abuses the procreative capacity of women to create and maintain unjust relationships between men and women. The reproductive capacity of a woman may be turned against her, and she may fall victim to oppression precisely because of this special ability of bearing and birthing offspring. In such systems, the (postulated or actual) specific characteristics labelled as female or feminine, including female sexuality, are underappreciated, degraded, repressed or entirely overlooked and abused, as well as being given mythical properties [24]. Control over female sexuality is connected to the patriarchal need to establish male control over women's fertility and reproduction on the one hand, and to the attempted control over women's gratification and enjoyment on the other, especially if such enjoyment is specific to women. In its extreme, the control of female sexuality is manifested in physical violence: the mutilation of female genitalia, rape (including marital rape and rape in war), brutal punishment of infidelity or sexual activity before marriage, etc. This not limited to violence practised by individual men over individual women; instead, these acts of violence are socially tolerated or even officially permitted as acts aimed at gaining power and consolidating power relations in a community [25].

6. Why women, and women in particular, need health care

Along with benefits for women (and women's health), sexual activity, pregnancy, labour, breastfeeding, menstrual and menopausal cycles also carry risks of a lower quality of life [10]. Half of humankind face specific health issues connected to the biological and sociocultural role of women as key for the proliferation of the species. These issues affect actual mothers as well as women who have no children due to social or personal circumstances. Some of these issues are an added burden on women's health; they may pose a health risk, restrict the maintenance and improvement of health or act as a hindrance to recovery; in extreme cases, they can cause illness, injury or death. Compared to men, women are particularly vulnerable due to their biological capacity in particular. Until recently, they risked their well-being and lives in ways that men did not due to unwanted pregnancies, complications during pregnancy or childbirth, consequences of miscarriages, abortions and other reproductive cycle events – in some places these risks are still significant. These are some of the key social conditions in which women live and which determine their worth, their standing in the family and the community, and their access to basic necessities, including education and health care. But women's sexual and procreative health is also threatened by sexual violence, sexually transmitted diseases, insufficient or inaccessible prenatal care and birth control, inaccessibility of safe abortions, and so on: despite modern social changes, women continue to face more hardship and limitations as regards their personal freedom than men.

In traditionalist historiography, medicine was given the role of saviour; medicine was portrayed as key in freeing women from the role of females who need to sacrifice themselves for the human kind to survive [26]. Due to the rise of contraceptives, safe abortion, and hospital childbirth, and the raising of popular awareness about sexual health, medicine has been regarded as a force that freed women from the risks of the unreliable and dangerous reproductive female body. It is a widely accepted belief that doctors are the only "true" experts on women's health, including sexual health, and that biomedicine is the key to improvement [10].

Globally, we strive to provide all women with optimal health care when they need it, and medicine plays an important part in this. Although medicine has undoubtedly accomplished much to maintain, improve and restore women's health and well-being, we cannot overlook its role in propping up women's unjust, subservient position in society, which is linked to reproductive capacity and sexuality in particular, as demonstrated above.

Do these types of discourse and practice contribute to liberation and the provision of free personal choice? Or do they instead restrict and regulate these, participating in decision-making on what is considered good and healthy as regards reproductive life, or risky, pathological or deviant as regards sexuality. As demonstrated by Turner, medical advice on how people should live may function as moral discourse to regulate bodies, control people's everyday life [27], and regulate the "quality" of populations – this is known as "biopolitics", the style of government that regulates populations by applying political power to various biological aspects of human life [28]. This type of medicine is particularly striking in fields like "public health", in measures to "promote health" or "a healthy lifestyle" for pregnant women, in organizing birth care, in the promotion or limitation of breastfeeding, in regulating how a mother should care for her child, in providing advice on how mothers should raise children, and so on [20, 29].

It must be stressed that when speaking of medicine, what is meant is not a monolithic structure, but rather a patchwork of complex dispersed processes, struggles, contradictions and inconsistencies; this has varying effects on the lives of people, depending on their gender, social status, age, and so on. We differentiate medicine as an institution with certain types of discourse and practice and health professionals. Among these professionals are individuals who may not always hold power, especially when they are women – midwives and nurses are often lower in the hierarchy than doctors, for example. On the other hand, being a woman does not always mean more equal cooperation with other members of health teams and empathy towards patients.

7. Medicalization

The concept of medicalization, as developed by Ivan Illich [30], is a useful tool in trying to understand the conceptualization of women's sexuality in the biomedical model of health and sickness; it provides space for a critique of the positivist side of medicine in an age of embodied culture [31-34], in which the body becomes the principal field of political and personal grievances, as claimed by Bryan S. Turner in his theory of modern society as a "somatic society".

Medicalization involves the identification or categorization of a certain feeling, state or behaviour as pathological, as something in need of treatment or intervention; it is a process in the course of which health or behavioural issues begin to be viewed, defined and treated as medical issues, a process in which everyday occurrences, phenomena or living conditions are reinterpreted as medical issues to be subjected to medical control and definitions emphasizing risks, pathology and the importance of intervention treatment or other types of "managing" or handling the issue. Health professionals, and doctors in particular, are the ones defining, studying and treating these issues. "Western" medicine, also known as allopathic medicine, which is supposed to be based on scientific findings, provides a rigorous framework in its many iterations to explain, categorize and classify a variety of symptoms and diseases affecting individuals. Health professionals use a number of different means to treat and prevent illnesses or alleviate health issues as well as improve people's quality of life. Let us not forget, however, that medicine has evolved in a certain conceptual framework like all other scientific fields, and is therefore based on implicit, often ill-defined and unclear presumptions, such as the concepts of masculinity and femininity, which is made apparent in fields like psychiatry, gynaecology and obstetrics; historically speaking, these are disciplines particularly employed as mechanisms of power, and their practices have widely been used to control and define normality, pathology and deviance [35]. Medicalization processes occur in different ways, such as through changes in social relations, the creation and use of language, the development of certain ways to solve problems while disregarding others, and the institutionalization of particular services while others are excluded. The consequences of medicalization include personal or social life decisions being made within a limited specific reference framework.

The expansion of medical authority into various fields has had important impacts on everyday life. Medicalization has become such a self-evident part of our lives that is takes significant effort to distance ourselves and listen to the facts.

Medicalization of individual areas of life does have its advantages. Medicalization can be critiqued in terms of medicine as a scientific authority and health professionals as experts, linking to questions about the control and regulation of individual groups or phenomena and the interplay between knowledge and power [18]. In analysing power relations, their complexity needs to be taken into account, as the issue of medicalization cannot be reduced to the desire to dominate certain areas of knowledge or its disseminators and the conscious need to regulate populations, even though these two factors are among its essential elements. If authority over the body/in the body, as Foucault suggests, is divided into the disciplining or individual bodies and the regulation of population, or biopolitics, both of these processes simultaneously occur at the same place in the context of controlling human reproduction – that is, on the female body, even *in* and *with* the female body. Maintaining subservience and control inevitably involves a certain degree of violence, which, however, may not always be visible or apparent on sight. Control employing physical force and corporal punishment, isolation and darkrooms frequently morphs into more subtle, yet equally effective tools, such as exposure to other people's gaze, coercion to self-monitoring, self-discipline and disclosure, and manipulation through feelings of obligation and guilt. What does "medicalization of female sexuality" mean, then, and what is the price paid by women, frequently without knowing why and for what purpose?

8. The medicalization of female sexuality and procreative activities

Over the past decades, a persuasive line of argument has been developed which allows us to look critically at the medical usurpation of childbirth and its control of obstetric care while noting both its positive and negative effects [22, 36-44]. Doctors have assumed essentially total control over the pregnant woman, for it has come to be expected to give birth in hospital, and so on. The focal point of our analysis is modern biomedical discourse in gynaecology and obstetrics, as well as selected institutional practices for pregnant women, women giving birth and women after childbirth, with a particular focus on female sexuality. The analysis delineates the extremes, limitations and trappings of the usurpation of female sexuality by medicine and draws attention to its internal contradictions, tensions and struggles.

Let us look at a few keys points. An important aspect of modernization is the regulation, management and control over the human body and sexuality in particular, and medicine has historically played an important role in these processes. Sciences and their application in medical practice are always established and formed within a certain social context, as proven by the historian of sexuality and the body Thomas Laqueur, who studied various conceptualizations of the body through sex differences in great detail. Inter alia, he drew attention to a particularly key shift from the uniform model of the human sexual anatomy in Europe in the 18th and 19th centuries to the dualist conceptual model of two sexes. One-sex theory conceptualized the human body as the same both in men and women – women have the same genitalia as men, only that female genitalia are on the inside rather than on the outside, meaning the only difference was superficial. Two-sex theory considered femaleness as permeating every cell of the body, meaning that the female body fundamentally differs from the male body [45]. This new conceptualization of the woman in medicine as the "other sex" resulted in positioning the female body as a separate entity. The emergence of gynaecology and sex endocrinology in the late 18th and early 19th century is linked to the dominance of a discourse practice in which sex and reproduction are more essential and determine women more greatly than men. Sexual anatomy and sexual differences were used to support the superiority of men over women. The subordination of women by men was based on hierarchical ordering of two different bodies and helped to establish a new understanding of gender with firmly defined roles. The one- and two-sex models and the victory of the latter over the former have been consolidated through their use in anatomy, gynaecology and practical diagnoses and treatment of women. According to Laqueur, no differences between male and female sexuality emerge in the one-sex model, and attention is drawn to the importance of female pleasure and orgasm in order to conceive, which later lose any visible role in the two-sex model, where the woman is designated a passive recipient of male active sexuality. Specific gender theories and gender differences or similarities are shaped in interdependence with social conditions, and the culture was the force which denied women the ability to experience sexual pleasure and gratification despite the already existing anatomical evidence about the role of specific female body parts and the importance of the clitoris.

In the 20th century Freud's theory about the vaginal orgasm, which replaced the adolescent clitoral orgasm and was a sign of a woman's maturation, and whose absence signified frigidity, turned out to be based on the two-sex model, which requires women to adapt their pleasure to their expected social role in spite of their bodily structure and neurology, rather than because of it. This theory, labelled "the cultural myth of the vaginal orgasm" by Laqueur, was followed by a number of male and female authors and made many women wonder about their inappropriate, infantile sexuality and undergo therapy.

After the Second World War, sexuality began to be studied empirically. American biologist Alfred Charles Kinsey published the Kinsey Report in two volumes, *Sexual Behavior in the Human Male* in the 1948 and *Sexual Behavior in the Human Female* in 1953. These findings were built upon in a confidential study at a St. Louis clinic carried out in the late 1950s by the American gynaecologist William Howell Masters to observe and empirically study the human sex act under laboratory conditions, along with his assistant Virginia Eshelman Johnson, who had no degree or official medical credentials. The pair carried out controversial studies about sexual experience in men and women. Their findings regarding female sexuality were relatively straightforward – almost all female orgasms are caused by direct or indirect stimulation of the clitoris. This empirically disproved Freud's theory about an "immature" clitoral and a "mature" vaginal orgasm.

What is important is to understand how particular knowledge is incorporated in mainstream discourses, medicine included, and used for normalization and control in the everyday lives of women. Medicine tends to commodify female sexuality. The emergence and acceptance of particular theories on female sexuality are linked to the social conditions of the time in which supposedly objective and independent scientific findings become a convenient tool to achieve goals not related to the wellbeing of individuals; at the same time, the conditions for the emergence and development of certain knowledge are themselves an intrinsic part of a certain reference frame of the dominant culture.

Medicine has contributed both to the improved sex lives of women and of their reproductive lives more generally; however, let us not forget its contributions to blaming mothers for a variety of social problems supposedly caused by inappropriate motherhood [20], ranging from various addictions to the increase in violence and the emergence of a narcissistic society [46].

Female sexuality has been pathologized with diagnoses like "hysterical" and "neurotic", and these so-called disorders treated in a variety of ways with differing levels of brutality; during the obsessive preoccupation with masturbation in the 19th century, even clitoridectomies were in use, among other methods, and contributions to reducing women to specific desirable and acceptable aspects were made by theories such as the concept of women's masochism [12].

Medicine facilitates the expansion of a market providing modern services modifying the female body to (socially) desirable norms, which women either voluntarily or involuntarily adhere to. For-profit medicine, with the express cooperation of physicians, markets absurd plastic-surgery procedures on the hymen, known as hymenoplasty or "re-virgination", which is problematic from an ethical standpoint. As long as a few drops of blood determine the value of women, women will be forced to undergo surgery to replace a potential "lost" patch of tissue with a couple of stitches. On the one hand, young women who live under specific religious or social norms regarding the "virginal", sexually "not-yet-tainted" female body, which is to belong to a particular man – often not of her own choosing – believe they need to undergo this procedure to protect themselves and their families. On the other hand, with every such procedure, medicine contributes to the perpetuation of "virginity", a construct affecting entire generations of women.

Other procedures promoted by the plastic-surgery industry include "vaginal rejuvenation", breast augmentation, facial cosmetic surgery, body-contouring surgery and facial procedures in the absence of any pathological condition, which are frequently, though not necessarily, based on the patriarchal idea of the sexual and sexualized female body as seen through the male gaze; this is at the very least controversial, if not outrightly upholding and consolidating the remnants of the patriarchal social order.

Currently, some branches of medicine also participate in the development of some ethically questionable new reproduction technologies, which have been proven to involve misuse and even abuse of women, like trafficking with eggs and embryos to offer commercial services of surrogate motherhood.

In history, discourses in medicine feature assumptions about the female orgasm, the lesser capacity of women to enjoy sex, or women's passive and men's active sexuality, as well as questioning of lesbian love and sex. Contrary to common (self-)perception, even today medicine is not neutral regarding sex expressions of gender and still participates in attempts to normalize certain sexual practices while pathologizing others, based on obsolete and disproven concepts – as seen in recent history in relation to the provision of access to infertility treatment for single women in Slovenia in 2001, for example. In public debate, those who opposed the proposed law problematized among other things the supposed motherhood of single or maybe homosexual women, where the sexual activity of a man is not desired or needed – with the support of some medical professionals.

8.1. Female sexuality and childbirth – The modern desexualization of childbirth

Female sexuality and its controversial links to medicine should be the focus of everyone dedicated to women's well-being, particularly during important transitions in life, such as puberty, childbirth and menopause. The medicalization of female sexuality is a phenomenon that affects women around the world and requires a detailed structured critique. As can be inferred from data obtained by studies, analyses of delivery-room procedures and available literature, the practices in modern obstetrics are frequently at odds with women's autonomy, ignore their feelings and knowledge and harm their bodies, mind and soul time and time again. It is part of a structural issue connected to the status of medicine, its position in the modern understanding and management of life, its power over transitions in life such as childbirth, the transfer of childbirth into the hospital, the use of specific prosthetic means to control life, illness and death, the "objective" and "legitimate" definitions of the normal and the pathological, the technologization of pregnancy, and the specific attitude to female sexuality.

This paper studies some of the types of medical discourse and practices in relation to the female gender, particular attitudes to female desire, pleasure and gratification that evolve with time, the control over reproduction, and the definition and construction of "good" motherhood.

How should we interpret the relationship between medicine and female sexuality, which is perceived as a gender-specific experience and practice in the life-cycles of ordinary women? We study the contributions of medicine to the everyday lives of women, which remain closely linked in many ways to caring for other family members and bringing the family into existence in the first place, that is, to the "production" and "reproduction" of people in general. In order to facilitate understanding of the issue of the medicalization of female sexuality as an important issue for midwives, quotes will be used below from archived statements made by women on their experience with care in maternity wards over the last decade – the testimonies were gathered by the author. This approach aims to facilitate greater awareness of the issue by using a research method that gives women a special position and is particularly esteemed in women's studies and feminist theory. Women's voices are heard and listened to, which is an important way of empowering women and one that may promote their contributions to thinking about cultural childbirth practices and their influence on the practice of perinatal care, which is supposed to be about helping and supporting mothers and their newborns.

Medicine aggressively participates in the development of new reproductive technologies and various practices which make parenthood possible despite any number of physical or medical obstacles – these are practices ranging from a variety of medically assisted conception methods to the overseeing of individual surrogacy procedures. Medicine's attitude to women, the female body and female sexuality is often full of contradiction; on the one hand, it assists women in achieving their goals or becoming a mother, while at the same time contributing to the exploitation of women's reproductive capacity by the privileged. Conception itself no longer requires sexual intercourse, and as specific knowledge and technology develops, medicine has begun looking into ways of reaching the phantasmatic goal of creating human life in a way that would eliminate the need for a female body to carry the child to term and give birth [47].

http://dx.doi.org/10.5772/60124

A special element of the medicalization of female sexuality, which this paper shall focus on, is the participation of medicine in separating motherhood from sexuality, excising female sexuality from childbirth and erasing the sexual component of the experience of giving birth. Paradoxically, the desexualization of childbirth functions as a component of control over female sexuality – that which is obscured or pushed aside and denied is just as important as that what is manifest or even excessive. The exclusion of certain knowledge and the link between knowledge and power is something to which Foucault has already drawn attention [28]. As noted by anthropologist Robbie Davis-Floyd, routine care for the mother at the maternity ward is so effective in masking the sexuality of childbirth that the majority of modern women are not even aware of the sexual character of childbirth [38]. It can be said that the culturally dominant image of modern childbirth has been "cleansed" of anything implying sexuality, and that any discourse involving a link between childbirth and sexuality is marginalized – what you would see in a typical birthing room is a woman in a hospital gown lying on a bed and covered with a sheet, looking more like a patient than an empowered woman giving birth to her child.

Let us take a closer look step by step. The entry of men into the process of childbirth as healers, medicine men and male midwives [40], which only expanded with the medical takeover of childbirth [48], also reopened questions about female sexuality. On one hand, this is interconnected with the need to control women's reproductive ability, while on the other, the idea of female sexuality as a threat to patriarchal order creates discomfort and anxiety and demands regulatory tools be developed. In light of this, some characteristics of the modern "design of childbirth" need to be reconsidered – including the institutionalization of childbirth, routine care and the implementation of certain procedures, such as the shaving of pubic hair, enemas, vaginal examinations and episiotomy, while foregoing others, such as nudity of the birthing women, body support and close contact between the birthing woman and her support network, the restrictions on audibly expressing labour pain and other feelings, pleasure included, and so on.

We can use a historical case to make the point. The emerging use of chloroform rather than ether to alleviate labour pain triggered a fight in the scientific community, which was detailed in the prestigious *Lancet* magazine. Some interpreted the "hysterical behaviour" of mothers in labour who had been given ether as an expression of sexual arousal, which was a threat to the obstetrician. According to certain medical opinions, labour pain merely masked sexual pleasure not requiring the involvement of a male. To prevent labour pain might then stop the mechanism neutralizing sexual arousal. A woman who is medicated to a pain-free state and whose sexual arousal is therefore unhindered regresses to an animal state and can no longer be controlled by a physician. This is the contradictory idea of the woman in the 19th century – is the woman primarily a sexual or a moral being; is she a seductress of men (doctors included) or a moral guiding light? The line of thought of the time, based on the two-sex theory discussed above, is easy to follow: the woman is a primarily reproductive being, meaning that her character is sexual, that is to say, animalistic; considering that the biologists of the time observed that animals were keen to copulate after giving birth, the idea emerged that childbirth could be a sexually arousing event for women. Physicians were suddenly trapped in their own contradictory (mostly unreflected) conceptualization of the woman. They considered the idea of "sexually aroused" women going through labour under anaesthesia to be "a danger to the patients, doctors and medicine in general". To assume as great a degree of control as possible, they recommended chloroform, which was to be administered in quantities that exceeded the dosage needed for mere pain alleviation. Anaesthesia during labour was approved not only to ease women's labour pain, but also to protect the physicians from unwanted reactions of the women in their care [19].

The current prevailing attitude to labour pain leads women to dissociate from physical sensations and pain as well as joy, pleasure and ecstasy. Some women, such as individuals recovering from sexual abuse, consider it vital to keep at least minimal control over the process of childbirth and dissociation is one way to achieve that, for example with effective medication to treat labour pain, such as epidural anaesthesia. Due to forgotten or at the very least incredibly marginalized knowledge about the integrity and interconnectedness of childbirth on the physical, mental and spiritual level and the physiological laws of labour, which (may) include both pain and pleasure, it is entirely understandable that many women consider the medical alleviation of labour pain to be a requirement, while seeing discussions about the internal power and capacity of the body to respond with its own way of alleviating pain as pushing women back to (ruthless) nature.

Assuming the vantage point of tension between pain and pleasure, intertwined during childbirth, let us think about how women experience usual childbirth practice in hospital with predetermined routine procedures. These have the woman lying on her back in bed, "hooked" on IV with induced and/or augmented contractions, with no constant midwife presence, making her feel that she has lost control of the situation and the procedures of the medical staff: she feels objectified – *"like being a walking uterus"* – and reduced to her physical body – *"I felt like a slab of meat"* – and has no say in what happens to/in her body: *"The doctor entered and without looking at me, pushed his hand inside of me, which hurt horribly, mumbled something and left."* Routine vaginal examinations are particularly revelatory, as this is the body part considered to be the most intimate of all. An interviewee recounts acts by the medical staff once she felt the need to push that she thought were wholly inappropriate. The medical staff carried out a vaginal examination, which she experienced as an act of violence: *"When the midwife called them over, they said, 'Impossible, it's impossible that she would be this dilated.' They go inside, 'Fantastic, fantastic, so soft, feel it, come and feel it.' They're just wriggling their hands inside of me! /the speaker is extremely distressed, note by Z. D./ Look at that, oh.'"* [49].

Ignorance about the interconnectedness of sexuality and childbirth is the consequence of induced amnesia, which, however, is not total and is visible, for example, in jokes made by doctors and sometimes midwives who act more like obstetrical nurses, at the expense of women – jokes they can make because of their status within the health-care hierarchy. For example: "It'll come out the same way it went in!" or "A woman of normal sexual health should enjoy childbirth a lot, considering that the child is so much larger than the penis" (as I find written in the notes I made during an interview with a Slovenian obstetrician in 1993). The problem lies in power relations; power is used to define how (if at all) female sexuality may be expressed at the maternity ward and to define what is normal and what pathological, and

http://dx.doi.org/10.5772/60124

frequently what is moral as well. That a specific medical idea of childbirth is prevalent in maternity wards is precisely why the idea that childbirth could be aided or labour pain alleviated with practices involving, for example, a woman stimulating her nipples or clitoris is unacceptable, and such advice is met with derision or disgust by health professionals. The problem is not that medical professionals are unaware of the effect of nipple stimulation on contractions, since understanding of this mechanism was the basis for the construction of a special device patented in the US to achieve stronger uterine contractions [50]. The device does not cause the same discomfort usually expressed by medical professionals when confronted with an explicit expression of female sexuality during childbirth, because it allows them to establish a distance. According to women's testimonies, as little as requesting perineal massage during labour, which can prevent rupture and injuries if applied gently, can meet with the disapproval of midwives in maternity hospitals. The medical approach to childbirth in modern hospitals is very much the "high-tech, low-touch" approach, in opposition to the "low-tech, high-touch" approach where understanding of the needs of women during birth includes the sexual aspect of the birthing process. Established ignorance about certain aspects of female sexuality and the potential for abuse is illustrated by a delivery-room case documented by the author, which involved the obstetrician "helping" the woman in labour during her vaginal examination by stimulating her clitoris without informing her beforehand or obtaining her consent; according to my personal notes, none of the experts moved in to stop this, acting rather as voyeuristic witnesses.

The desexualization of childbirth was also significantly advanced due to the relocation of childbirth into institutions, which largely occurred in the second half of the 20th century; this involved the creation of a new norm stipulating that women should give birth in a hospital setting, and the forcible enforcement of this norm – despite current efforts to expand the choice of childbirth settings. This shift was initially presented as an important factor for maintaining the good health of women and children and the prevention of illnesses and death, while overlooking or disregarding the effect of institutionalization on the process of childbirth, the lack of privacy, the failure to provide certain aspects of care and the introduction of new routine procedures as well as the increased participation of men in a field where technology and routine procedures are given priority. What emerged was a desexualized female body in labour, shaven, genitals exposed, exposed to a controlling gaze and authoritarian touch, while ignoring sexual content, forbidden expression or care that would evoke the institutionally undesirable sexual aspect of childbirth; this, too, is an important vantage point from which the consequences of the framing of the maternity ward, with professional care provided by the public health-care system, as the mandatory childbirth setting, need to be examined.

The issue of desexualizing childbirth is multi-layered – childbirth is more difficult when women are forced to disassociate from what their bodies are telling them and bow down to a procedure imposed from the outside, when they have to ignore their own expression and sounds and control themselves in order for the professionals to find their behaviour acceptable. It is especially ironic considering that the institutionalization of childbirth was intended to provide higher-quality birth care. The routine use in hospitals of artificial oxytocin, which induces contractions and/or stimulates them, may be interpreted as an anticipated response to the conditions of childbirth in an institution where the logic of the natural progression of childbirth is devalued or even ignored. Physiological childbirth is on one level based on a sensitive, changing hormone cocktail in the birthing woman and baby, and is closely connected to the well-being of the woman and child. If we obstruct or hinder otherwise functioning patterns, external interference becomes a necessary replacement for the physiological dosing of oxytocin in birth care that places the woman at the centre and respectfully supports her – this becomes more likely to happen outside of an institution. In contrast to authentic midwifery [51], taking natural body responses into account is not a strength of modern obstetrics, and staff, both doctors and medicalized midwives, frequently interfere and express a sense of hurry – or even, completely inappropriately, impatience. One example from data collected in an Internet questionnaire about birth experiences in Slovenia in 2005: *"What bothered me the most was that the staff kept saying, 'Come on, ma'am, everyone else gave birth already!"* [49]. In order to understand the basic needs of women during childbirth, we need to find a gender-specific understanding and sensibility and then develop appropriate approaches. Authors who acknowledge the interconnectedness of childbirth and sexuality compare the usual conditions under which we have sex, which provide intimacy, a relaxed environment and the knowledge we are not under anyone's control, with the conditions for successful childbirth, which are exactly the same: privacy, a warm, darkened space, no control or comments on appearance or behaviour. It is clear that pressuring your partner to have an orgasm will almost certainly have the exact opposite effect; similarly, scolding and expressing disapproval of a woman and her partner for kissing while she is in labour is only going to hinder the process, as often remarked by Marsden Wagner, a medical dissident who dedicated his work to supporting the well-being of mothers and babies and supporting autonomous midwifery [52].

Women need their individual course of pregnancy and childbirth to be respected, with the lowest possible degree of interference and forced adherence to routine; they do not wish to be told to hurry up or slow down, as corroborated by modern studies of childbirth physiology – childbirth is optimal when interference and intrusive procedures are the fewest. What is more, it has been proven that women and children benefit hugely from the presence of support networks and staff who deliberately try to be as non-intrusive as possible in order to allow the individual to relax and let the natural progress of childbirth take over. It must also be taken into account that every individual mother has her own particular way of giving birth, and she must be offered support, which includes adapting the setting. If individuals are able to relax and focus on giving birth, they will find it easier to listen to their own body, which in turn makes the midwife's job easier and more fulfilling. The degree of restrictions and expectations imposed by medical staff on women in labour, especially regarding her physical expression, is illustrated by another example from my notes of a consultation with a mother of a newborn in 2011, who bared her breasts during childbirth and was subsequently scolded by the midwife, *"Put your clothes back on, will you, this is not a beach."*

Ensuring privacy is one of the important aspects of a birth setting. Individual women have differing definitions of privacy. However, the feeling of one's privacy being limited definitely has no positive effects on childbirth; too many people in the delivery room, unknown personnel performing care, having to disclose personal information or even undergo a physical examination, even a vaginal examination, in the presence of others, e.g., during the rounds in post-natal wards, etc., are all intrusions on privacy. It should be kept in mind that, rather than being irrational, the institutional bans or restrictions on the presence of people the mother-to-be feels close to – her partner, other supportive women or doulas – are based on the understanding of power and control over the woman in labour and her freedom, and on the expectation that she must conform to the social expectations imposed by the institution during birth.

The widespread practice of episiotomy during typical childbirths is a classic example of a specific conceptualization of the female gender and her body in obstetrics, which is based on doubts over the capacity of the female reproductive system to deliver a baby without harming it. A decade ago, episiotomies were performed in over 50% of vaginal births in Slovenian maternity wards [49]. Episiotomy has adverse short-term and long-term consequences – more bleeding, pain, vaginal deformity – and affects women's sex lives both mentally and physically. Scientific data on when an episiotomy is justified show that an acceptable rate of episiotomy that would not increase the number of injuries in women and babies would be about 10%. There are midwifery practices with significantly lower rates of episiotomies or even none, but the disassociation from the sexual dimension of childbirth in modern obstetrics is made abundantly clear by the generous use of the procedure. One cannot help but agree with authors who have labelled the practice "sexual mutilation of women" [53].

9. Conclusion

If modern obstetrics does not rethink and expand its ethical principles, it will continue to deliver inhumane treatment to women – ignoring their needs, objectifying them, marginalizing their sexuality during the birthing process, and taking their power and control over a situation where these are of the highest importance. The challenge before us is to instigate a shift towards cooperation between birthing women, midwives and doctors. Midwifery is considered a caring profession, where midwives provide care to each woman and child individually during pregnancy, childbirth and early motherhood. The core tenet of midwifery is its positioning on the side of the woman; today, midwifery is undergoing modernization and it is therefore vital to recall what we have learned about the medicalization of female sexuality. Having reviewed the discourse and practices in which many midwives in institutions participate and perpetuate, we must call for more awareness about the midwife principle in modern society. We cannot ignore the question of midwives' (dis-)comfort with female sexuality, and the importance of understanding this as well as the connections with procreation capacities. Physiology and culture, which permeate every woman, her personal history and family traditions, continuously fluctuate and seek balance. Are we, as women, sufficiently self-aware that we know what we and our counterparts need in order to be able to say yes or no with a degree of responsibility to ourselves and others during childbirth, as in intimate relationships which include sexual activities?

We are still searching for answers to questions regarding, for example, the price women pay for (a semblance of) reproductive freedom. What has liberation won for us or taken away as regards sexuality? Why do women partake in this? How do women fight back? Is there a way of moving past the medicalization of women's physiological sexual and procreative processes that we can embrace now and in the future? We all have to ask ourselves how to exist in a woman's body; we must be brave in taking on questions, empowering each other and working together to create opportunities to make our personal freedom a reality. To carry out decisions, to use our brain and not let others decide about important aspects for us. To stop definitions from limiting us. To dare to see, think and know in order to live well and work well, and, most importantly, to do good.

Author details

Zalka Drglin*

Address all correspondence to: zalka.drglin@guest.arnes.si

Women's Studies and Feminist Theory, Slovenia

References

[1] Gerhard J.F. Desiring revolution: second-wave feminism and the rewriting of American sexual thought, 1920 to 1982. New York: Columbia University Press; 2001.

[2] Allyn D. Make Love Not War: The Sexual Revolution, an Unfettered History. New York: Taylor & Francis; 2001.

[3] Brownmiller S. Against Our Will: Men, Women and Rape. New York: Simon & Schuster; 1975.

[4] Rich, A. Of Woman Born: Motherhood as Experience and as Institution. New York: Norton; 1986.

[5] The Boston Women's Health Book Collective. Our Bodies, Ourselves for the New Century. A Book by and for Women. Toronto, Ontario, Canada: Touchstone Books; 1998.

[6] Starčević G. Volk v supermarketu: antropologija ustrojenega sveta. Ljubljana: KUD Apokalipsa; 2011.

[7] Vance C., editor. Pleasure and Danger: Exploring Female Sexuality. Routledge: Boston; 1984.

[8] Carnes P. Out of the Shadows: Understanding Sexual Addiction. Center City, Minnesota: Hazelden; 2001.

[9] Shorter E. Written in the Flesh: A History of Desire. Toronto, Ontario, Canada: University of Toronto Press; 2006.

[10] Doyal L. What Makes Women Sick. London: Macmillan Press; 1995.

[11] Blank H. Virgin: The Untouched History. New York: Bloomsbury Publishing; 2008.

[12] Shorter E. Women's Bodies: A Social History of Women's Encounter With Health, Ill-health, and Medicine. New Brunswick, London: Transaction Publishers; 1997.

[13] Knibiehler Y. Histoire des mères et de la maternité en Occident. Paris: Presses Universitaires de France; 2000.

[14] Fox Keller E. and Longino H.E., editors. Feminism and Science. Oxford Readings in Feminism. Oxford, New York: Oxford University Press; 1996.

[15] Jacobus M., Fox Keller E. and Shuttleworth S., editors. Body/Politics. Women and the Discourses of Science. New York in London: Routledge; 1990.

[16] Jordanova L. Sexual Visions, Images of Gender in Science and Medicine between the Eighteenth and Twentieth Centuries. New York: Harvester Wheatsheaf; 1989.

[17] Turner B.S. Regulating Bodies. New York: Routledge; 1992.

[18] Foucault M. The Birth of the Clinic: An Archaeology of Medical Perception. London: Tavistock; 1973.

[19] Poovey M. Uneven Developments. The Ideological Work of Gender in Mid-Victorian England. London: Virago; 1989.

[20] Oakley A. The Captured Womb. A History of the Medical Care of Pregnant Women. Oxford: Basil Blackwell; 1986.

[21] Martin E. The Woman in the Body: A Cultural Analysis of Reproduction. London: Open University Press; 1989.

[22] Tew M. Safer Childbirth? A Critical History of Maternity Care. London: Chapman and Hall; 1988.

[23] Harding S. Whose Science? Whose Knowledge? Thinking From Women's Lives. London, Milton Keynes: Open University Press; 1991.

[24] Kristan Z. Materinski mit: kultura, psihoanaliza, spolna razlika. Ljubljana: Založba Delta; 2005.

[25] Chantal L., Hauser M. Nicht aufhören anzufangen. Zürich: Rüffer&Rub Sachbuchverlag; 2008.

[26] Borisov P. Ginekologija na Slovenskem od začetkov do leta 1980. Ljubljana: Slovenska akademija znanosti in umetnosti; 1995.

[27] Turner BS. The Body and Society. Explorations in Social Theory. London: Sage; 1996.

[28] Foucault M. Vednost – oblast – subjekt. Ljubljana: Študentska založba; 1991.

[29] Drglin Z. Rojstna hiša. Kulturna anatomija poroda. Ljubljana: Založba Delta; 2003.

[30] Illich I. Medical Nemesis. London: Calder and Bryers; 1975.

[31] Gallagher C. and Laqueur T., editors. The Making of the Modern Body: Sexuality and Society in the Nineteenth Century, Berkeley, Los Angeles, London: University California Press; 1987.

[32] Gallop J. Thinking Through the Body. New York: Columbia University Press; 1988.

[33] Apple R.D., editor. Women, Health, and Medicine in America. A Historical Handbook. New Brunswick in New Jersey: Rutgers University Press; 1992.

[34] Braidotti R. Nomadic Subjects. Embodiment and Sexual Difference in Contemporary Feminist Theory. New York: Columbia University Press; 1994.

[35] Canguilhem G. The Normal and the Pathological. New York: Zone Books; 1991.

[36] Adams A.E. Reproducing the Womb: Images of Childbirth in Science, Feminist Theory, and Literature. Ithaca, New York: Cornell University Press; 1994.

[37] Campbell A. Childfree and Sterilized: Women's Decisions and Medical Responses. London: Cassell; 1999.

[38] Davis-Floyd R. Birth as an American Rite of Passage. Berkeley, Los Angeles, London: University of California Press; 1992.

[39] Ehrenreich B. and English D. For Her Own Good: 150 Years of the Experts' Advice to Women. New York: Anchor Books; 1989.

[40] Donnison J. Midwives and Medical Men: A History of Inter-Professional Rivalries and Women's Rights. New York: Schocken Books; 1977.

[41] Goer H. Obstetric Myths versus Research Realities. A Guide to the Medical Literature. Westport, Connecticut, London: Bergin and Garvay; 1995.

[42] Rothman B.K. In Labor: Women and Power in the Birthplace. New York: W. W. Norton; 1991.

[43] Scully D. Men Who Control Women's Health: The Miseducation of Obstetrician – Gynecologists. Boston: Houghton Mifflin; 1980.

[44] Spallone P. Beyond Conception: The New Politics of Reproduction. London: MacMillan Education; 1989.

[45] Laqueur, T. Making Sex: Body and Gender from the Greeks to Freud. Cambridge: Harvard University Press; 1990.

[46] Lasch C. The Culture of Narcissism. London: Abacus; 1980.

[47] Corea G. The Mother Machine: Reproductive Technologies from Artificial Insemination to Artificial Wombs. New York: Carper and Row; 1985.

[48] Davis-Floyd R. and Sargent C.F., editors. Childbirth and Authoritative Knowledge: Cross-Cultural Perspectives. Berkeley, Los Angeles, London: University of California Press; 1997.

[49] Drglin Z., editor. Rojstna mašinerija: sodobne obporodne vednosti in prakse na Slovenskem, Koper: Univerza na Primorskem, Znanstveno-raziskovalno središče, Založba Annales: Zgodovinsko društvo za južno Primorsko; 2007.

[50] Google Patents. Method for inducing uterine activity through nipple stimulation. http://www.google.com/patents/US4794915/ (accessed 10 December 2014).

[51] Gaskin I.M. Ina May Gaskin's Guide to Childbirth. New York: Bantam Dell; 2003.

[52] Wagner M. Pursuing the Birth Machine. The Search for Appropriate Birth Technology. Camperdown: ACE Graphic; 1994.

[53] Wagner M. Episiotomy: a form of genital mutilation. The Lancet 1999; 9168 1977-1978.

Towards Unprejudiced Midwifery Care — Midwifery Students' Views on Homosexuality

Barbara Domajnko

Additional information is available at the end of the chapter

http://dx.doi.org/10.5772/59116

1. Introduction

Through history and across different social and cultural contexts, homosexuality was and still is presented as a sin, a disease, a crime, or a variation of sexual orientation. Following pressure from strong activist movements, the American Psychiatric Association removed homosexuality from its official diagnostic manual in 1973. In Slovenia, the Criminal Code treated homosexuality as a criminal act until 1976. WHO eliminated homosexuality from its list of diseases in 1991. Nevertheless, misinformation and prejudiced views strongly persist in certain areas, the most discussed currently being same-sex families and the right of gays and lesbians to adopt children. Common, general, and erroneous assumptions that get replicated in public discourse are, for example: homosexuality is not normal/natural; it is impossible to have two fathers or mothers; and it is for the good of the children to prevent their adoption by gay or lesbian couples, to name just a few [1]. These assumptions reflect the prevailing heteronormativity [2], which denormalizes and excludes all other variations of intimate practices and thus regulates our relationships, attitudes, expectations, and behaviour.

More than ever before, homosexuality today is understood in socio-political terms, as a question of social (in)equality. Attention is focused on socially excluding practices; that is, practices that deprive certain people of their basic rights, resources, and opportunities in a society. From the perspective of social psychology [3], these discriminatory practices are grounded in social categorization. The formation of stereotypes involves simplistic generalizations and neglects individual specifics. Stereotyping thereby uncritically overstates typical characteristics of a group at the expense of an individual's unique character. Stereotypes are, furthermore, value loaded. Stereotypical negative claims, usually formed even before coming into contact with the person or group talked about, are called prejudiced judgements. Since they are negative, they are related to behaviour excluding certain groups of people from the core of the society and relegating them to its margins. The core society, or "us", is considered normal, righteous, and just, while the margins, "them", are attributed a negative, abnormal, and endangering character [4]. Applied to sexuality, heterosexuality is considered a norm (hence the term heteronormativity), pushing homo, bi, and transsexuality to a marginal position. Marginalization is justified and naturalized (presented as natural) in several ways, but it is grounded in prejudiced presentation of certain social minorities as endangering the majority [2]. Although it seems to make little sense, dominant discourses employing different representational strategies to depict certain minorities in negative ways, persistently and powerfully persuade the majority to recognize these minorities as a threat and to act defensively.

From the sociological perspective, the relation between expressed attitudes and real life behaviour is not straightforwardly cause-consequential but rather complex [5,6]. LaPiere's famous study was carried out in 1934 in the United States of America when anti-Asian feelings prevailed. He travelled with a Chinese couple around the country and they were only turned down once out of 251 times, when they asked for a room in a hotel. Later, he sent mail survey to the same hotels and 92% of the respondents claimed that they would not serve Orientals. Prejudices attitudes, therefore, could not simply be taken as predictors of discriminatory behaviour. What had to be taken into account were wider situational social factors. In face-to-face contact, especially, less discrimination was detected. Generalization of the causal relation therefore proved problematic, and the importance of different intervening social and personal variables that were activated when an individual person encountered a unique social situation were stressed. Similarly, considerable problems with defining attitude as a concept appeared. It was established that attitudes were not underlying stable entities but rather varied according to circumstances. Further complexity regarding the distinction between verbally expressed attitudes and their latent constellation was pointed out. Also, presupposing that behaviour could change only if attitudes changed first, neglected the power of social structure to affect behaviour. The latter proved an even greater determinant of behaviour than attitude. Martin Luther King Jr. is often quoted in this respect: "Morals cannot be legislated, but behaviour can be regulated. The law cannot make an employer love me, but it can keep him from refusing to hire me because of the colour of my skin" [6]. It is very important to pass laws prohibiting discrimination. It is of equal importance to then implement them systematically and persistently.

It may seem then that actions speak louder than words, but comparing the two would only be to engage in endless discussion about which is more powerful and influential — actions or words. Instead, we should change the perspective and focus on the interpretation that actions manifest through words. We shall adopt this view by observing the changing manifestations of discrimination. Researchers [7,8,3] distinguished between the old and new forms of racism. Slavery and apartheid, for example, were explained in terms of biological inferiority, brutally enacted in direct physical contact as explicit hatred and violence. People were physically segregated. In such forms, racism was condemned — transparent expressions of racism are now globally socially unacceptable. Racism itself, however, was not rooted out. It transformed into the new type, which presents itself in democratic lights and denies being discriminatory. It claims to be a defender of the majority's rights that are endangered by minorities claiming to be deprived and fighting for more privileges. New racists avoid direct contact; rather, they keep their distance from their targets. The new racism is symbolic and cultural. Instead of manifest aggression, it deploys a more indirect and covert strategies such as passive decline and ignoring the minorities. The transformation to more subtle and indirect manifestations established a much stronger relationship between attitude and behaviour. Symbolic racism is primarily a discursive racism. Discourse is a concept that helps us to understand language use within its social context, as a specific form of social interaction [9]. Within a social constructionist perspective we not only understand the world as we can describe it through language but we actively (re)create it by making different interpretations of it — texts and talks are, therefore, social practices [10]. Interpretations differ in descriptions and values. For example, there is a great difference between descriptions of a bruise as a consequence of a fall and a push. Contrary descriptions can be used to describe and value the same physical event, but which create two different interpretations with completely different judgemental values, and social and personal consequences — the event can be interpreted as an accident or an act of violence, respectively. Our reality is a discursive one and it is important, and far from coincidental, who possesses the power to interpret, whose version of the world is taken to be the correct and true one.

The power of discourses is also enabled by structural conditions of dissemination. The basic means of disseminating information today is provided by media of mass communication. People learn more about what is happening around them and in the world from mass media than from their personal experience; their knowledge is therefore mediated through media discourse. As such, media should be the prime locus of our critical attention. Critical discourse analysis developed out of that understanding and need [9,11,12]. Critical discourse analysis of Slovenian mass media texts on homosexuality [2] reveals five basic homophobic strategies: stereotypization, medicalization, sexualization, normalization, and homosexuality as a secret. Discriminatory discourse nowadays is rarely straightforwardly aggressive and explicit, but the same exclusionary effects remain. Some scientists claim its effects are even stronger, because symbolic discriminatory discourses present themselves as democratic, normal, and common sense, something we need not doubt and be critical about. Hate speech nowadays avoids direct disregard; rather it subtly discredits, humiliates, disrespects, and deprives people of dignity. As such, it is no less discriminatory than the older method. Understanding language use as discourse helps us surpass the distinction between actions and words — it stresses doing (discriminating) by using words (interpreting certain people as less worthy). That is why modern activists fighting inequality also operate at the level of legislation, and strive to enforce laws on hate speech. In Slovenia, freedom of speech is written into the Constitution, yet its Article 63 also prohibits the encouragement of inequalities, spread of hatred, intolerance, violence, or war. The Criminal Code was enacted in 2008; article 297 regulates hate speech and article 141 prohibits discrimination on the grounds of sexual orientation.

Surveys on public opinion in Slovenia detected homophobia. The great majority of the respondents did not personally know any people that were homosexually oriented yet more than half of them would not want a gay or a lesbian to be their neighbour [13,14]. In another study [15] more than half of included gays and lesbians had experienced violence due to their homosexual orientation: 90% characterized it as psychological, 24% as physical, and 6% as sexual violence. It was mostly caused by strangers and enacted in public places (61%), but to a lesser extent also by parents (25.8%), relatives, friends, and school peers (25%). At work, 4% suspected they had been fired due to the disclosure of their sexual orientation. Regarding family planning, 42% of gay and lesbian respondents wished to have a child and 40% did not. It was interpreted as reflecting their understanding of an unfavourable social context and scarce chances they were given to realize this wish, which therefore mainly stayed repressed. These data also indicated the (large) extent of deliberation they invested in this question, given that their wish for a child is often considered to be selfish and without any consideration for that child.

Children of gay and lesbian couples are stigmatized and victimized: that is, attributed the role of the victim from the outside by the prejudiced wider society, not based on their own bad experience or objective data of poor living conditions. It is supposed to be for children's own good not to have same-sex parents, although in most cases one of the partners is a biological parent of a child, making such prejudice an instance of homophobia dressed in altruistic clothes. Namely, there is no evidence of lower quality parenting in gay or lesbian couples. Children do not report problems if the relations within the family are of good quality. Rather, the problems appear once they enter an institution or society at large, where others start telling them that they are different or less worthy. Only then do children become at risk of homophobia, discrimination, and violence. Compared to activist attitudes and the demonstrative silence of gay/lesbian parents and their children in Sweden and Germany, the Slovenian response is to hide — they were afraid of being abused. Homosexuals do have children, either from their previous heterosexual relationships, by in vitro fertilization, or some other kind of arrangement. Rainbow families already exist but they are excluded at the symbolic, legal, and social levels [16].

Social inequalities do not refer only to the economic, political, and cultural conditions of life, but also manifest in health. In the last two decades, WHO has been strongly promoting the awareness of the social determinants of health, especially in terms of the devastating effects of health inequalities [17]. The social determinants of health are defined as economic and social conditions that influence the health of people and communities, and are shaped by policy choices, power, money, and resources that people have. This also means that they could and should be decreased by appropriate socio-political action. Research showed that homophobia and discrimination — negative (pre)judgements, hatred, and practices that deny social participation or human rights — have negative effects on (mental and physical) health of the discriminated and the accessibility and quality of health care services provided to them [18]. Health problems of lesbian, gay, bisexual, and transgender (LGBT) people have only just recently begun to be surveyed [19]. They were found to have worse mental health than the general population, they were more likely to commit suicide, and they had a higher rate of alcohol consumption and misuse of substances/recreational drugs and related problems. They had higher rates of physical ill health, worse self-reported health status, more acute physical symptoms, and chronic conditions. It is important to understand that this morbidity is caused by psychosocial stress stemming from stigma and discrimination coming from the wider society but also occurring in healthcare settings. On the one hand, health professionals were reported to have denied homosexual people access to certain services, excluded them from decision making. or made inappropriate comments. On the other hand, health professionals were experienced as not being knowledgeable about homosexuals' lifestyle and specific health care needs [20]. Studies showed that homophobia amongst health professionals had negative consequences for the care of lesbian and gay clients [21,22]. This is also one of the reasons why LGBT people keep their sexuality a secret from health care professionals or even fail to engage with health services. A general ignorance of lesbian needs is not only present in the field of health care but also social services [21]. In Slovenia, such a deficit combined with homophobic standpoints was already detected in the field of social and consultant work related to mental health, where evidence was found that homosexuality was still considered to be a disorder [23].

2. Problem and aim

Health care professionals and their respective professional fields are a part of society and thereby prone to be affected by various public discourses and policies. It is a constitutive part of their supportive, therapeutic, and educational work to include and empower people in their endeavour to promote, preserve, or restore health. Their professional ethics require them to be knowledgeable, objective, and non-judgemental, and to provide equally accessible and high quality services to all. Midwives are among the health care professionals that deal most directly with different aspects of human sexuality. One of their important competences, therefore, is to gain knowledge and develop sensitivity towards different forms of (health) inequalities related to sexual orientation, starting by becoming aware of and overcoming their own prejudices.

The aim of the original study was to study attitudes of first year students of different health professions towards homosexuality and homosexual parenting. The focus of this chapter is placed on midwifery students. Right at the start of their studies, the students were not yet exposed to a faculty professional curriculum. The purpose was to get an idea of the extent and types of potential prejudices against gays/lesbians and homosexual parenting. On these grounds, it will be possible to revise and adjust the contents of existing study programmes to provide knowledge supporting equal midwifery care in the future. Another aim was to raise awareness of a special discourse pattern — the disclaimer — which in today's' society, especially, effectively supports the hidden persistence of all sorts of prejudices, while giving the illusion of tolerance in the speaker.

3. Methods

A qualitative study was designed and carried out. It involved the first year students of different study programs at the Faculty of Health Studies (University of Ljubljana) at the beginning of the school year 2013/2014. The participation of students was voluntary, free from any pressure, and anonymous. They were informed of the aim of the study and given enough time to ask for additional information. They were asked to provide descriptive answers to eight open ended questions regarding their conceptualization of sexuality in general, sexology as a science and its relevance to their professional field, and their attitudes towards homosexuality and same-sex parenting. They wrote their answers on a piece of paper. Textual material was generated from 49 students of occupational therapy, 16 of orthotics and prosthetics, 39 of radiologic technology, 36 of sanitary engineering, 28 of nursing, and 29 of midwifery. Their answers were typed into an electronic format, and then coded and analysed using a critical discourse analytic framework [9,11]. Acknowledging the purpose and theme of this book, the primary analytic attention was attributed to the answers of midwifery students. In particular, the analysis focused on disclaimers.

In democratic societies, social norms prescribe tolerance and prohibit prejudice and discrimination among citizens. Speakers breaking this social norm by expressing negative opinions against certain individuals or social groups, therefore, need to apply denials or at least some form of mitigation strategy to maintain positive self-presentation in public. A disclaimer enables this impression management. According to van Dijk [7], a disclaimer (an apparent denial) is a specific structure of language use, the prototype being: "I have nothing against them, **but**...." In the first part of the structure, a generally tolerant attitude is stated while the second part continues with a specific negative opinion. This structure does not support inference from specific to general and as such presents a defensive strategy against potential accusations of socially unacceptable intolerance. On the other hand, the denial is only apparent, because the specific disregard is nevertheless inconsistent with the prevailing social norm. What is negatively stated is not really denied, at least not completely. Rather, the speaker wishes to deny the possible negative inferences about his social intolerance and to establish positive self-presentation. The tolerant attitude is left unsupported by evidence that the speaker really does not have anything against them. At its best, it therefore expresses limited social acceptance.

Billig [24] claimed that the social value of not being prejudiced is so general and deep-rooted that is also shared by the most extreme political agents. The disclaimer represents an advanced justification against the accusation of being prejudiced. It is not merely public impression management. Speakers also justify themselves to those who hold similar values and to themselves. It is therefore also a discursive strategy of self-justification: by the self to the self.

The analysis focused on disclaimers, through which prejudiced viewpoints against gays, lesbians, and same-sex parenting were identified. Results are presented by excerpts from direct writing collected from the midwifery students that participated in our study. Each excerpt is labelled with a code in brackets, where M stands for midwifery and the number for a random number attributed to the study participant. Excerpts are grouped under several sub-headlines according to themes that appeared to be most prominent.

4. Results and interpretation

Among midwifery students, 12 of 29 were supportive of gays and lesbians in all aspects of their lives, 10 expressed prejudiced opinions against homosexual couples having the right to get married and especially to adopt children, and seven struggled in forming a clear standpoint on the matter. In comparison to the first year students of other programs participating in our study, the ratio of supportive answers was quite high. Their positive attitude was related to the ethical principles of (post)modern societies — accepting and respecting diversity:

I accept homosexuality, I treat it equal to heterosexuality, which I believe is the only appropriate way of thinking in a modern society. (M3)

I accept them, they do not bother me. We are not all the same, I accept differences. (M17)

Homosexuals are completely common people, the same as heterosexuals. We all have the right to choose a partner at our own will. (M13)

My attitude to homosexuals is positive as I have two friends who are homosexuals. I can talk to them practically about everything. I have never scorned them and I never will. They are people just like us. (M15)

All of our respondents were aware of the social norm prescribing the same rights and treatment for all citizens, and consequently condemning discrimination. That is why homophobia was rarely explicitly stated; in all 29 cases of midwifery student answers, it appeared only once:

Personally I do not approve of homosexuality. I believe it is some sort of a mistake (in thinking, genes, development of a human being), as it is not natural. (M4)

On the other hand, the responses of those who expressed some sort of disregard or did not yet form a clear opinion on that matter, were full of disclaimers. Two different patterns were recognized. Intolerance was either disclaimed within a single sentence or across larger meaningful instances of talk:

*They do not bother me, **but** I avoid them (if I can). (M19)*

*I have nothing against them. I am tolerant to people different from me. If somebody is a homosexual, it does not bother me. **But** I do think they expose too much in public. That is why they are often laughed at or attacked. (M23)*

Before we tackle the topic at hand in greater detail, we shall consider student opinion on sexuality and midwifery in general from a broader perspective. From this context, we shall then return to our respondents' attitudes towards homosexuality

5. Sexuality

Mostly, the students agreed that in Slovenia sexuality persisted as a taboo topic in public discussions. In their opinion, the older generations still found it very difficult, even inappropriate, to talk about it publicly, while the younger generations were becoming much more relaxed and ready to discuss it among themselves and in public. Also, in their opinion sexuality was related to health. They not only explained this relation in terms of pathology and sexually transmitted diseases, they often defined it as a vital human need and an element of happiness and quality of life. In broader terms, they explained it as an intimate relation between two people who loved and cared for each other, which means they also took consideration of partnerships in terms of a much wider perspective. Focusing on the intercourse, they stressed:

Sexual intercourse with the right person relaxes, which bears influence on wellbeing, means less stress. (M5)

It is known that during sexual intercourse the hormones of happiness are released. Our body is more relaxed and at the same time it is a type of physical exercise and contributes to our health. (M19)

These aspects become very important when interpreting standpoints expressing negative attitudes towards homosexuality and the rights of homosexuals. If sexual relations with the partner of one's own choice can have such positive effects on a person's health and wellbeing, why is it acceptable for heterosexuals but not homosexually oriented people? Standpoints against homosexuality do not only deprive a group of people of the free choice of a sexual partner, but also prevent them from the positive effects of sexuality and partnership on their health, wellbeing, and general quality of life.

Although society at large, in the opinion of our respondents, was becoming more relaxed and open, sexuality was still considered to be a fairly intimate matter. Even the younger generation was not always willing to discuss it seriously and frankly with anyone. As one of the students said, she was more likely in public to exaggerate, make things up, and present herself in a more socially favourable light. For the practice of midwifery it is important to stress that in the opinion of one of our respondents, some people also considered health professionals (potentially also midwives) as strangers, that is, people they did not feel able to discuss their sexuality with completely openly and frankly:

I can talk about it quite relaxed with friends and my partner. But I feel uncomfortable to discuss it with strangers (a nurse at gynaecologist). (M18)

On the one hand, therefore, sexuality is perceived as a highly intimate matter, but on the other hand, it also exposes the influence on public health and is a topic of public discussions and political action.

6. Midwifery

Midwifery students included in our study expressed their understanding that midwives were involved in the most intimate and vulnerable aspects of the lives of women and couples:

Midwives "enter" the intimate sphere of human beings. (M4)

A midwife deals with the intimacy of a woman in her most frail moments. (M8)

It is therefore of utmost importance to establish a safe and trustworthy relation:

Our work reaches to the very intimate sphere. It is up to us, how to approach the intimacy, in what way, showing respect. (M22)

Midwives affect the lives of women, couples, babies, and families. Our respondents enumerated the facts that midwives give advice and teach about, for example, good relations in partnerships, sexual practices, the safety of intercourse, contraception, problems related to sexuality, family planning, healthy pregnancy, sexuality during pregnancy, labour, and parental roles. Knowing and understanding the type of partnership is a precondition of their work. Our respondents were aware that it was therefore important to respect the sexuality of women and couples they came into contact with in order to be able to provide relevant and high quality information and midwifery care.

7. Homosexuality

The presentation of the students' standpoints and attitudes towards homosexuality is divided into several thematic parts. First, the established distinction between public and personal opinions is illustrated and interpreted. Several adverse judgements were found, the most controversial among them being related to homosexual parenting. The analysis then focuses on different defensive strategies our respondents used in trying to avoid giving the impression of being discriminatory. The most common justification strategies to keep an apparently tolerant social demeanour despite expressed disregard were: the necessity of parents of different sexes, the social exclusion of children of homosexual parents, the questioned normality and naturalness of homosexuality, and the perception of homosexual orientation as a voluntary and conscious decision. The revealed tensions testified to the complexity of expressed attitudes towards homosexuality, which was further illustrated by reported feelings of being caught in contradictions among social norms, public opinion, and personal attitudes.

7.1. The society is discriminatory — I am not

Almost all respondents agreed that society at large persisted in being very negative, prejudiced, and discriminatory towards homosexuals, although they judged that the overall situation was becoming more tolerant. A common strategy of denying their own homophobia was to attribute it to others. At least that looked convincing at the beginning of their talk; as it continued, the disclaimers helped to reveal much more prejudiced talk than the speakers were ready to admit:

I personally do not mind, but I know a lot of people who do mind very much, even though I do not know why. Everyone should live as they want. I think the most important thing is to be happy and if that makes them happy, that is fine. But I do not agree with homosexual parenting because I would not want to be a child of two mums/dads. (M10)

In my opinion most of the people still look at homosexuals in a different way — in a way as if something was wrong with them, in a mocking way... I have no comments against the homosexuals. Everyone has the right to decide, choose their partner. But regarding homosexual parenting, my standpoint is that it is inappropriate, as homosexual partners cannot raise a child. (M16)

In both cases, the speakers started by establishing a difference between others that disregard homosexuality and themselves, who were not bothered by distinctions in sexual orientation. They even elaborated their views by acknowledging some basic human rights: everyone should live as they want, everyone has the right to be happy, and everyone has the right to make their own decisions. At least that was what they believed in principle. Right after that, a discursive turn followed: in their opinion, homosexuals, unlike heterosexuals, did not have the right to decide they wanted children and attain happiness through parenting. The speakers thereby set limitations to these universal rights and freedoms of people with homosexual orientation, which was very much in contradiction with their alleged tolerant attitude and much closer to the homophobia they attributed to others.

7.2. Citizens with limited rights

As illustrated above, there are still areas of social life where the apparently universal rights and freedom of certain individuals or groups of people clearly end. In our respondents' opinions, homosexually oriented people did not have equal opportunities in today's society, mainly when searching for employment, but they did not agree with that injustice. On the other hand, they identified several types of behaviour that were completely unproblematic for heterosexuals but perceived as endangering their heterosexual identity when observed with homosexuals:

I have no problems meeting a homosexual couple; they as well are just humans. But I believe they should be a little bit more reserved when showing it in public. (M19)

They do not bother me personally until they wish to have children. (M8)

In most cases, our respondents were personally bothered by the public appearance and disclosure of homosexuals, even if it was just holding hands. Some of them objected to homosexual marriages. The most controversial topic of all, however, proved to be homosexual parenting.

7.3. Homosexual parenting: the social exclusion of children with two mums or dads

Some midwifery students were supportive of homosexuals in all aspects of their lives, including parenting. They grounded their opinion in their belief that characteristics of good parenting were not related to sexual orientation, and stressed the importance of a child's personal satisfaction and wellbeing:

I support homosexual parenting. I believe homosexual parents can offer equally warm shelter (if not more) as heterosexual ones. (M3)

I support them if they decide to have children as they too have the right to create their own family. (M7)

I am not prejudiced. It is important that the child feels well. (M9)

I have nothing against the adoption of a child by homosexual partners, as a child needs love and care and for that you do not need different sexes. The inner side of a human is important. (M12)

Parents of the same sex could also raise a child appropriately. Also, not all heterosexuals are suitable for parenting and cannot take this responsibility but their pregnancy is not controlled. I do not believe the sex of parents is so important for raising a child. The missing role of a father or a mother could be taken up by somebody else, other relative. (M18)

If the parents are OK, I do not see any problems. A lot of children have a father and a mother, but they experience violence or something similar. I think we should ask children how they feel (for example when asked by schoolmates about their mother or father). If they do not mind, neither should we. (M20)

They do not have the same rights, but they should, for example, two homosexuals could raise a child better than parents if there is alcoholism, quarrelling or violence present in the family. (M21)

I believe a child should grow up in a loving family, traditional or some other, as sometimes living with a father and a mother that do not take good care of their children is worse than with two loving mothers. (M26)

Regarding today's' society and events that are reported on radio and TV, I think sometimes homosexual partners could offer a child a better life than parents that have no consideration of when to have a child. (M28)

Not all students were so straightforwardly supportive. Aware of the potential accusation of intolerance, our respondents' arguments involved quite complex justifications for their prejudiced and discriminatory views. Several times, the inappropriateness of homosexual parenting was backed up by a claim that a child needed parents of both sexes:

I am not bothered until they wish to have children. In my opinion a child needs a man and a woman. (M8)

I don't consider it appropriate that some children would have two mums and dads. (M5)

Literally speaking, a child cannot have two mothers or two fathers, at least if we understand these terms in their traditional, biological sense. Raising and taking care of a child, however, is also or even primarily a socio-cultural phenomenon, which is not unconditionally related to gender, blood ties, or the number of persons involved. The key question in this discussion therefore seems to be: is sexual orientation related to the ability to be a good parent? As one of the respondents, expressing her supportive standpoint towards homosexual parenting, noticed:

Sexual orientation is not the only thing that defines a man. (M19)

Once we deconstruct the misunderstanding of parenthood in purely physiological terms (as an ability to conceive a child), it becomes clear that social acceptability or appropriateness (who is allowed to take care of a child) is a quite different question. Instead of focusing on the economic/material, socializing, and protective aspects of raising a child, it is frequently turned into a political question that has also been on the public agenda in the past, when laws were discussed and passed regarding adoptions, foster care, and in vitro fertilization, to name just a few.

The second identified strategy used to justify prejudiced claims was intertwined with the first one, and referred to the presupposed negative reaction of society, social exclusion, and victimization of children:

I don't consider it appropriate that some children would have two mums and dads. Such children would probably be excluded from the society. (M5)

Although I said that I have nothing against these persons, I do not agree that they could adopt children. I think it could influence their lives because the Slovenians are still much closed and we do not know how to accept difference and a consequence would be that such a child would be mocked (mockery depression suicidal thoughts). (M14)

Although I hold no prejudice towards homosexually oriented people, I consider homosexual parenting unacceptable because of the child, who would be exposed to mockery and rejection. (M27)

Mockery and rejection by society were mentioned several times in combination with the perception of homosexual parents as two mums and dads as the terms themselves, stressing the biological aspect of parenting, alluded to their very inconsistency. Prejudiced and discriminatory society was frequently (mis)used as an argument for depriving a certain group of people of the opportunity to establish a family instead of recognizing the urgent need to promote tolerance and acceptance of differences. The most extreme instance of this line of thought can be illustrated by the following excerpt in which the speaker explicitly acknowledged that homosexual parents could even be more loving than heterosexual ones, before drawing a negative conclusion:

Homosexuals do not bother me personally, although if I see something like that in the street, it looks strange, because I am not used to it, but it does not bother me. Of course they have the same rights as the rest of citizens; I believe that sexual orientation should not influence human rights. But I do not consider homosexual parenting to be appropriate. Otherwise they can be even more loving as normal parents, but mainly from the child's perspective, I do not think it is appropriate. (M11)

According to this excerpt that claimed to speak in favour of the child, it was more important to conform to prejudiced social attitudes than to allow the child to be raised by loving homosexual parents. Was this speaker really not bothered personally by homosexuals and convinced that they had the same rights as heterosexuals? The speaker was no expert on homosexual parenting and was repeating prejudiced and superficial judgements about homosexual parenting in general. It was an act of discursive discrimination, because such judgements, not supported by any sound evidence, still have social consequences. Namely, they perpetuate still further the prejudiced social talk that is usually attributed to others and so easily disclaimed by the speaker. Our respondents referred to this public opinion (the society, the others) as very influential in many excerpts. Who, then, is the one that really objects to homosexual parenting? As another midwifery student noticed, social disregard of same-sex parenting is today's reality, but the key question promoting tolerance should be: who is the society? Who creates social relations? Is it them or is it us, perhaps even me?

I believe that many homosexuals would care for a child better. Homosexual parenting is not problematic for me, I support it. Society is the problem — we teach our children that homosexuals are different. If we didn't then the children of homosexuals would not be condemned by their peers. (M15)

Changing public opinion is not a new phenomenon. Life is a process involving constant change and one commonly attended by rejection of that change. The social exclusion once experienced by children born out of wedlock is now happening to children in rainbow families and will continue to happen to children of another marginal social group in the future. It is important to recognize that exclusion is never determined by nature or the children themselves but by social relations and the attitudes of adults, by norms reflecting social power.

The third identified type of justification of prejudiced and discriminatory talk was found in the interpretation of homosexuality, homosexual partnerships, and/or parenting as abnormal and unnatural. This can, again, be done fairly straightforwardly (that is, explicitly stated), or implicitly alluded to (inferring difference from a "normal" couple or family):

They do not bother me personally; it is not their fault that it is happening to them. But it gets on my nerves that they would have equal rights as couples (marriage, adoption of children) as I do not think it is natural. (M2)

My opinion is relative to the matter. As a friend I do not have any problems, but I would personally have to think very hard if it was a very important decision to be made, for example adoption of a child by a normal or homosexual couple. I would prioritize a normal couple as I think every child has the right to live in a normal family, not in a family that is not accepted by the society. (M22)

It is a common but erroneous belief that "normality" is a property of nature and that both categories exist irrespective of their social context. From the discursive perspective, normality and nature are both social constructs — something is not "normal" or "natural" in and of itself, it is interpreted as such within discourse. Following this line of thought, attention should be put on the speaker's constructions. Instead of claiming that something is normal or natural, a critical thinker should be attentive to what is normal to whom, and to ask according to whose criteria is something is deemed natural? Interpretation is related to the social position and power of the speaker. Abnormality of homosexuality exists only in heteronormative societies.

The fourth strategy apparently justifying the speakers in expressing discriminatory claims was identified in our respondents' conception of sexual orientation as an individual's conscious decision. Within this perception, homosexually oriented people voluntarily decided against the prevailing social heterosexual norm and were thus themselves intentionally challenging society to accept them. Following this line of thought, it is homosexuals themselves who should take the blame and responsibility for the consequences that follow from such socially unfavourable decisions:

They have certain rights, but not all, for example the right to adopt children, as it was their own decision to be different, not able to conceive a baby. (M8)

I see no sense in homosexual orientation, but I think it is a personal decision of each individual and that is why I have no prejudice towards these people but there appear many doubts when such a couple wishes to adopt a child, because a child could have problems... We all know that it takes a man and a woman to create a new life. Who intentionally decides against this must accept also the facts that follow as a consequence. (M27)

The same principle of social responsibility for one's own decisions is followed also in contrary cases:

I accept homosexuality; a man on his own cannot influence his sexual orientation. (M1)

I think they are completely normal people like the rest as they do not have any influence over their orientation. (M19)

People not having any say in or power over the phenomenon were also not to be blamed and punished for the (unintended) consequences. They deserve our sympathy and support.

7.4. Torn between social norms, public opinion, and personal attitudes

It has become evident from the excerpts so far that the current debate about homosexuality involves many contradictory aspects. On the one hand, the prevailing social norm is tolerance and the reduction of inequalities. On the other hand, the alleged public opinion is still very negative and, although dispersed and intangible, very strong and influential. Civil movements are quite active but marginalized. This leaves many people bewildered and wandering among different discourses: the traditional attitudes they were socialized into, and their own experiences and critical observance of the society they live in. For our respondents, it was sometimes really difficult to form a clear personal standpoint:

Although I do not want to accept them differently, I keep a certain distance towards them. (M5)

I do not yet have a clear opinion on homosexual parenting. I have not thought about it thoroughly, but I feel inclined to think that everyone should have the right to have children, irrespective of their sexual orientation. (M1)

I think the important thing for a child is to have loving parents, but it is also true that children today do not yet understand difference and would probably experience much harm from their peers. (M19)

I have not taken sides yet. On the one hand I do not support it because of the children, on the other hand I support it because the child and this relationship can be more sound and the child more loved as in certain partnerships... A child should have a mother and a father, but a homosexual couple can love a child very much and a child can grow in a loving environment. (M23)

Homosexual parenting — why not? Better two mums than none or a careless one. But I think that the public is not ready yet and a child would suffer the consequences in the end. (M25)

As we learned from sociological research, it is not enough to study attitudes and expect that by changing them, we will automatically change behaviour; it is necessary to simultaneously change social structures:

I object to homosexual parenting and adoption, because of the child and the society, but I will accept it, if such law will ever be passed. (M24)

My opinion towards homosexual persons is not really formed — sometimes it bothers me more, at other times not at all. It is difficult to describe my attitude, mainly because the public opinion is at many occasions clearly stated (that it is not right). (M26)

The real name of the game therefore seemed to be striving to represent oneself positively to others as well as to themselves. Even when personally tolerant, our respondents felt pressed to conform to what they detected was (negative) common sense as the prevailing public attitude. To mitigate disregarding standpoints and make them conform to the highest social norm of respecting differences, they (we?) learned to apply various justification strategies in order to defend from potential accusations of intolerance.

8. Discussion

The respondents in our study were the future providers of health care. Many of them expressed very tolerant and well-supported views. On the other hand, analysis also identified prejudiced and discriminatory standpoints towards homosexuality. It is therefore important to include the deconstruction of common prejudices in health care curricula. They should include knowledge of the roots and consequences of homophobia. Identification of prejudiced talk and instances of discrimination should be followed by open critical discussion, which should result in the weaker presence of prejudices and thereby, hopefully, fewer inequalities in health.

This discourse analysis showed many different types and instances of prejudiced standpoints against gays/lesbians, and especially their families, among the first year students of midwifery. The ratio of supportive answers among midwifery students compared to their colleagues from other programmes was relatively high, yet less than half were supportive in all respects. In general, students interpreted sexuality as a human intimate need that was positively related to a person's health and quality of life if the partner was chosen according to their preferences. By rejecting homosexuals, they therefore deprived gays and lesbians of this basic right and need. The respondents who expressed their negative attitudes towards homosexually oriented people proved that sexual orientation was not only a personal but also a social matter, the latter having influence over the former. It became evident that choosing the partner of one's own preference was acceptable only within socially accepted heterosexual norms. A code of ethics binds the professional to be objective and apolitical. Professional curricula should therefore also address these topics to enable midwives to become aware of the discriminatory attitudes and norms, and to provide non-discriminatory care.

In the views of our respondents, midwifery spanned private and social spaces. People usually find it difficult to reveal and discuss their private matters with others. Midwives could be experienced as strangers. An important professional question, especially in cases of socially unfavourable sexual practices and relations, was how to develop sensitivity to a person's discomfort and vulnerability, establish a safe, respectful environment, and build trust. Our respondents claimed that midwifery provided a women-centred care. Besides acknowledging individuality and respecting the rights and dignity of a person, this also brought to the fore the question of client involvement. Namely, it is not enough to care for the clients' health and their needs, the clients themselves should be supported to express their own experiences, needs, and preferences. Caring professions should not only provide care but also empower clients to take an active role in decision making related to their care [25].

It was seen from our respondents' answers that homophobia was easily attributed to others and rarely identified in the self. Through the analysis of apparent denials, it was nevertheless found that even students that claimed to be tolerant considered homosexuals as citizens with limited rights. Gays' and lesbians' rights to live as they chose was partly accepted, but tolerance mostly ended when the question of parenting came to the fore. The rejection was explained in terms of social discrimination and victimization of children. Four sub-themes were identified: a child needs parents of both sexes; society rejects same-sex families and victimizes the children; homosexuality is not normal and natural; (homo)sexual orientation is a conscious decision of an individual. We shall address them respectively below.

In Slovenia today, the proportion of families composed of a married couple with children is dominant, but has been on the decrease ever since 1991. In 2011, the ratio of single parent families increased to 25% and the ratio of unmarried couples with children to 10.8%. In the same year for the first time, the national statistical office recorded the ratio of reconstituted families (defined as families composed of two partners with children, where at least one child is not a biological child of both partners) as 4.1% [26]. Other sources estimate the ratio of reorganized families is much higher, around 30% [1]. Statistics about different types of social parenting (especially homosexual parenting) are difficult to obtain and are currently very dispersed, largely because people do not feel comfortable and safe to disclose data about their private lives for the fear of stigma and social exclusion. There is no doubt, however, that many different types exist in growing numbers that cannot be neglected or pushed to the margins. Using terms and numbers alluding to blood ties (two parents; a mother and a father) is therefore primarily a way of naturalizing and normalizing only one of the many existent family relations and thereby implicitly stigmatizing and excluding all the rest.

Social parenting is established in opposition to a blood related conception of parenting. It is primarily focused on care and is as such defined as a social-emotive and intimate relation between an adult and a child that involves economic responsibility and is constant in temporal terms [27]. Blood relation is not unconditionally related to the quality of parenting. The quality of a family is related to the quality of relations and processes within it — such as taking care, taking responsibility, showing respect, enabling a sense of self-worth, allowing autonomy, providing means, and support and security — rather than to its form or structure [28,1,29]. Furthermore, contemporary conceptualizations of the family stress the prime importance of the subjective, lived judgements of people over structural, blood, or legal ones [28]. It is therefore important how family members feel about, treat, and take care of each other, factors not determined by the blood that circulates through their veins.

Society rejects gay and lesbian families, although the usual argumentation follows a paradoxical pattern. Commonly, the exclusion is explained in terms of the harm done to the children, which is said to come from the unfavourable social surrounding itself. The discriminatory society is therefore taken as an argument for not letting gay and lesbian couples take care of children instead of being criticized for being discriminatory. The discrimination of society is thereby sustained instead of challenged. Namely, the same people who accuse society are its very components; they themselves could therefore make a difference and be tolerant. As Urek

[28] said, accusing society of being immature only acknowledges and perpetuates discrimination but does not contribute to any changes.

In Slovenia, studies [1,28] identified and rejected the following common arguments against gay and lesbian families in Slovenia, all referring to the care of children: children have difficulties in developing their sexual identities; children have more behavioural and personality problems; they are victims of discrimination due to their parents' sexual orientation; and they are forced to live in same-sex families. According to Golombok [30], children living in single parent families or with social parents (homosexual partners included) from their earliest age showed no more psychological distress than peers from more conventional backgrounds. They had the same positive self-esteem and were considered by their peers to be good friends. The most emotionally stressful experience for the children was not having same–sex or social parents but in witnessing hatred and abuse. According to research, children of same-sex families were happy, intellectually successful, and tolerant [31]. Golombock [30] also proved that the presence of a father (or a mother) was not necessary for the development of sexual identity. Biological parents were considered a prototypical constellation for the development of a child, but children living with a single parent or social (homosexual) parents developed their sexual roles equally well. A comparison of children of homo and heterosexual families showed no difference in their sexual identity; children of homosexual parents formed their sexual identity without any confusion. The negative effects of single parenting had to do with the negative socio-economic consequences of a divorce: that is, poor economic conditions (if separation was related to diminished social standard) or small social networks and support received by them. If a single parent was well situated and had a large social network, no differences from other children were detected. On the contrary, some reported closer and warmer contacts, which reflected in life satisfaction. The important risk factor in any family type, therefore, was the lack of trust and good communication. All children face problems and dilemmas when growing up. They can all experience rejections and discrimination of some sort, due to their weight, figure, or some other physical characteristic; behaviour; or family arrangements they live in. It is difficult to avoid such negative experiences, but children can be supported in overcoming them. Good quality family life therefore depends on what is going on in the family, not who belongs to it.

It was interesting to observe the persistence of arguments related to normality and nature despite existing evidence that homosexuality had existed in different regimes and cultures at approximately the same ratio throughout history, regardless of social attitudes. Due to varying definitions and favourability of the social context, it is very difficult to calculate exact numbers. The commonly accepted data originate from Kinsey, the famous researcher of sexual behaviour; he claimed that each society included approximately 10% homosexual people [15]. Same-sex behaviour was also documented as a nearly universal phenomenon in animals, across species, from worms to frogs and birds, and it was further discussed how it had also contributed to the evolution of the species [32]. From the sociological perspective, it is soundly argued that what is established as normal (in opposition to pathological) is at each point in time defined by culture and ideology rather than being grounded in nature [33]. Presuppositions that heterosexuality is natural, normal, and right, thereby marginalizing other orientations and practices as unnatural, abnormal, pathological, and wrong, is one of the basic tenets of heteronormative ideology/discourse/society.

Also, the analysis identified misconceptions about sexuality as a conscious decision. Science has not yet provided its final answer on the origins of homosexuality. Research spanned across various topics, but none has managed to prove the existence of a homosexual gene, specifics in the structure of the brain, or any other physiological differences. Social factors also did not prove to be able to change sexual orientation, they only made people suppress or deny it. Today, homosexuality is understood as a variation in human sexuality [15]. Gays and lesbians themselves typically do not think that they voluntarily chose their sexual orientation and heterosexuals would probably claim the same.

Our respondents' reporting to be torn between the social norm of tolerance, discriminatory public opinion and their own more tolerant attitude could be interpreted as a sign of society's development. It proves the plurality of opinions, but also their competing powers. It is important to support this process by providing places and times for discussion within workplaces, professional education programmes, and public places.

Implications for midwifery already documented in the literature are vast and manifold. For the purpose of inciting further systematic research and study, we shall only briefly outline key areas: the clients' perspective, the midwives' perspective, and the students' perspective. Starting from acknowledging the client perspective, there are many qualitative studies giving voice to lesbians. A study on lesbian parents' experience of antenatal care, childbirth, and postnatal care identified the extensive presence of heteronormative communication, which was experienced as embarrassing for the participant parents as well as for care providers [34]. There is evidence of positive experiences of lesbian women during pregnancy and childbirth. Lesbians, however, also raised worries about postnatal care, parent education, and the structure of the patient records with no place for the female partner. They stressed that confirmation of parenthood was important, especially for the co-partner. In a study of experience of care provided during their partner's pregnancy, childbirth, and the postnatal period [35], the co-mothers' message was that they felt treated like everyone else, but not quite. They pointed out the need for acknowledgement, need for care designed to suit same-sex couples and the need for midwifery staff to recognize co-mothers as an equal parent of the child [36]. The least discussed topic seems to be midwifery acknowledgment of their role in supporting gay parenting. The needs of two men searching for information and possibilities to start a family, attend parental training, and receive good care [37] remains to be put on the professional and political agenda. Our respondents enumerated that midwives give advice and teach about good relations in partnership, sexual practices, the safety of intercourse, contraception, problems related to sexuality, family planning, healthy pregnancy, sexuality during pregnancy, labour, and parental roles. How many of these tasks, and in what aspects, relate to a male gay couple?

Evidence exists that health care outcomes for lesbians improved when health care providers were knowledgeable about and sensitive to the unique needs of lesbian clients [38]. It is of utmost importance to the lesbian's health and specifically to the outcome of labour, potential post-natal depression, and bonding with the baby, for example. The key question arises [21]:

how well equipped are midwives to provide effective and appropriate midwifery care to them? Following that finding, guidance for health care providers in supporting the childbearing lesbian couples was prepared on the basis of literature overview regarding lesbian experiences. Four areas of concern were identified: disclosing sexual orientation to caregivers and finding lesbian-sensitive caregivers, considering options of conception, assurance of partner involvement, and legal considerations related to the protection of both parents and the child [38].

There are many barriers that midwives themselves identified within their current practice. Wilton [21], in her discourse analytic study, documented the following five themes: anxiety about sexual difference, fear of female sexuality, the sexualization of lesbianism, the characterization of lesbianism as "sick" or "unnatural", and an inability to identify lesbians with any certainty. According to Jackson [39], many midwives fell into a conceptual trap stemming from reducing lesbians solely to their sexual orientation: namely, that they did not come into contact with lesbians because by the very nature of their sexuality they could not become mothers. They also made heterosexist and erroneous assumptions about pregnant women being in a sexual relationship with a male. It was repeatedly evidenced in inattentive heterosexist use of language: for example, referring to a father instead of a partner or an important supportive other. It led to malpractice, where lesbians were ignored and left invisible in midwifery care. Many midwives saw the positive side and described the lesbian love-relationship as strong and caring, but also detected their vulnerability stemming from their being different. It was important for midwives to acknowledge their own attitudes and culturally sensitive non-verbal communication, as well as considering the co-mother's needs and role as different compared to those of fathers. Although caring for lesbian couples was seen as unproblematic, midwives described experiences of ambivalence or anxiety in the encounter and they had noticed that some couples had negative experiences with maternity care [40]. The theme is also gaining grounds in Slovenia. Božnar, in a review of foreign literature on lesbian motherhood [41], aimed to motivate midwifes to consider the topic. In the relation of the midwife towards a lesbian, her partner, and their baby she stressed the importance of knowledge, understanding, and respect for lesbian mothers and their partners. Another important practical concern and research topic is homosexuality among midwives. A literature review showed little relevant literature on lesbian, gay, bi, and transsexual midwifes in the UK. The lack of their recognition carried personal and organizational implications, as it was supposed that homophobic attitudes negatively affected also their acceptance at the workplace [42].

Research also focused on future health care professionals. Jones [43] in a study of attitudes of higher education students in health profession educational programs showed high levels of discomfort when working with lesbians or gays. The majority of them believed their study programme had not adequately dealt with this issue. It was also one of the main results of our study that students found the topic relevant to their field of expertise and expected their study program to equip them with relevant knowledge. Regarding their unique position in the health care system (the field of sexuality and reproduction), midwives therefore need to know how to establish a safe environment for a lesbian to "come out" to the midwife and the knowledge to understand and support the patient's lesbian lifestyle. Midwives should become knowledgeable about lesbian culture and sexuality, learn to use nonheterosexist language, be non-judgemental, to raise awareness, and reject socially constructed prejudice [39]. This should also involve the visibility of homosexuals in informational material on sexuality, family planning, pregnancy, labour, parenting and partner support, and midwifery.

9. Conclusion

Homophobia is neither inevitable nor universal. It is socially constructed and maintained through homophobic discourse. Discourse is a powerful means of inciting and perpetuating prejudiced and discriminatory talk at the more implicit levels of communication. Disclaimers proved powerful discursive strategies of impression management. Their structure is such that it enables the speaker to express prejudiced attitudes, yet keeps the facade of tolerance. Language use perceived in its social context goes beyond mere articulation, it involves simultaneous action. Constructing and maintaining prejudices and discriminatory talk about homosexually oriented people may also result in unequal health care. Evidence was collected from gays and lesbians, midwives, and midwifery students. Gaining knowledge helps us overcome prejudice and fight discrimination. Understanding the powers of discourse gives us tools to deconstruct discriminatory messages and practices, triggers our critical thinking skills, raises our awareness, and enables us to act more tolerantly. Knowledge about homosexually oriented people and their health needs empowers health care professionals to provide better and more equal health care. In Slovenia, research should systematically be deployed to provide knowledge on LGBT people and their health needs, and professional education programs should adequately address them to deconstruct prejudices, raise awareness of discriminatory practices, and thus enable midwives to provide relevant, emphatic, holistic, and equally accessible midwifery care.

Author details

Barbara Domajnko*

Address all correspondence to: barbara.domajnko@zf.uni-lj.si

University of Ljubljana, Faculty of Health Sciences, Ljubljana, Slovenia

References

[1] Švab A, Urek M. Nove partnerske in družinske oblike — primer istospolnih partnerskih zvez in družin v Sloveniji. V: Rener T, Sedmak M, Švab A, Urek M. Družine in družinsko življenje v Sloveniji. Koper: Založba Annales; 2006. p127–50.

[2] Kuhar R. Medijske podobe homoseksualnosti: analiza slovenskih tiskanih medijev od 1970 do 2000. Ljubljana: Mirovni inštitut; 2003.

[3] Ule M., editor. Predsodki in diskriminacije: izbrane socialno-psihološke študije. Ljubljana: Znanstveno in publicistično središče, 1999.

[4] Leskovšek V., editor. Mi in oni: nestrpnost na Slovenskem. Ljubljana: Mirovni inštitut; 2005.

[5] Duckitt J. Prejudice and Behaviour: A review. Current Psychology: Research and Reviews 1992/93; 11(4): 291–307.

[6] Chaiklin H. Attitudes, Behaviour, and Social Practice. Journal of Sociology and Social Welfare 2011; 38(1): 31–54.

[7] van Dijk TA. Discourse and the denial of racism. Discourse and Society 1992; 3(1): 87–118.

[8] van Dijk TA. New(s) racism: A discourse analytical approach. In: Cottle S. (ed.) Ethnic minorities and the media. Buckingham: OUP; 2000. p. 33–49.

[9] Fairclough N, Wodak R. Critical discourse analysis. In: van Dijk TA (ed.) Discourse as Social Interaction. London: SAGE; 1997. p. 271–80.

[10] Potter J. Representing reality: discourse, rhetoric and social construction. London: SAGE; 1996.

[11] van Dijk TA. Critical Discourse Analysis. In: Schiffrin D, Tannen D, Hamilton HE. The Handbook of Discourse analysis. Massachusetts: Blackwell Publishers; 2008. p. 352–72.

[12] Erjavec K, Poler Kovačič M. Kritična diskurzivna analiza novinarskih prispevkov. Ljubljana: FDV; 2007.

[13] Toš N et al. Vrednote v prehodu II (Slovensko javno mnenje 1990-1998), Ljubljana: FDV, CJMMK; 1999.

[14] Toš N. et al. Vrednote v prehodu III (Slovensko javno mnenje 1999-2002), Ljubljana: FDV, CJMMK; 2004.

[15] Švab A, Kuhar R. Neznosno udobje zasebnosti: vsakdanje življenje gejev in lezbijk. Ljubljana: Mirovni inštitut; 2005.

[16] Zaviršek D, Sobočan AM. Mavrične družine grejo v šolo. Ljubljana: FSD; 2012.

[17] Marmot M, Wilkinson RG, editors. Social Determinants of Health (2nd ed.). Oxford: OUP; 2006.

[18] Pascoe EA, Richman LS. Perceived discrimination and health: a meta-analytic review. Psychological Bulletin 2009; 135(4): 531–54.

[19] Edwards J. The healthcare needs of gay and lesbian patients. In: Kuhlman E, Annandale E (eds). The Palgrave Handbook of Gender and Healthcare. Palgrave Macmillan; 2012. p. 290–305.

[20] Fish J, Hunt R. Prescription for change. Lesbian and bisexual women's health check. London: Stonewall; 2008.

[21] Wilton T. Towards an understanding of the cultural roots of homophobia in order to provide a better midwifery service for lesbian clients. Midwifery 1999; 15(3): 154–64.

[22] Experiences of healthcare 2012. http://www.stonewall.org.uk/documents/experiences_of_healthcare.pdf (accessed 21 August 2014).

[23] Urek M. Vodič za preživetje skozi socialno-varstvene službe ter službe duševnega zdravja za lezbijke in geje. Socialno delo 2002; 41(2): 113–8.

[24] Billig M. The Notion of 'Prejudice': Some Rhetorical and Ideological Aspects. Text 1988; 8: 91–110.

[25] Hermansson E, Mårtensson L. Empowerment in the midwifery context — a concept analysis. Midwifery 2011; 27(6): 811–6.

[26] Gospodinjstva in družine, Slovenija, 1. Januar 2011 — končni podatki. http://www.stat.si/novica_prikazi.aspx?id=4029 (accessed 21 August 2014).

[27] Zaviršek D. Med krvjo in skrbjo: Socialno starševstvo kot širitev koncepta starševstva v današnjem svetu. Socialno delo 2009; 48(1–3): 3–16.

[28] Urek M. Lezbične in gejevske družine v Sloveniji: implikacije za socialno delo. Družboslovne razprave 2005; 21(49-50):155–74.

[29] Švab A. Sociološki vidiki fenomena novega očetovstva: primer očetovstva in starševstva v lezbičnih družinah. Teorija in praksa 2007, 44 (1–2): 142–58.

[30] Golombok S. Parenting: What really counts? London, New York: Routledge; 2000.

[31] Zaviršek D. Gaybyboom v Sloveniji. Narobe 2008; 2(5): 21.

[32] Bailey NW, Zuk M. Same-sex sexual behavior and evolution. Trends in Ecology & Evolution 2009; 24(8): 439–46.

[33] Lock M. Accounting for Disease and Distress: Morals of the Normal and Abnormal. In: Albrecht GL, Fitzpatrick R, Scrimshaw SC. (eds.) Handbook of Social Studies in Health and Medicine. London: SAGE Publications Ltd.; 2000. p. 259–77.

[34] Röndahl G, Bruhner E, Lindhe J. Heteronormative communication with lesbian families in antenatal care, childbirth and postnatal care. Journal of Advanced Nursing 2009; 65(11): 2337–44.

[35] Larsson A-K, Dykes A-K. Care during pregnancy and childbirth in Sweden: Perspectives of lesbian women. Midwifery 2009; 25(6): 682–90.

[36] Erlandsson K, Linder H, Häggström-Nordin E. Experiences of gay women during their partner's pregnancy and childbirth. British Journal of Midwifery 2010; 18(2): 99–103.

[37] Gay-Friendly OBs, Midwives, and Doulas in NYC. http://itsconceivablenow.com/gay-friendly-obs-midwives-and-doulas-in-nyc/ (accessed 21 August 2014).

[38] McManus A, Hunter LP, Renn H. Lesbian Experiences and Needs during Childbirth: Guidance for Health Care Providers. Journal of Obstetric, Gynecologic & Neonatal Nursing 2006; 35(1): 13–23.

[39] Jackson K. Midwifery care and the lesbian client. British Journal of Midwifery 2003; 11(7): 434–7.

[40] Spidsberg BD, Sørlie V. An expression of love – midwives' experiences in the encounter with lesbian women and their partners, Journal of Advanced Nursing 2011; 68(4): 796–805.

[41] Božnar R. Babiška nega lezbičnih mater. Obzornik zdravstvene nege 2010; 44(1): 33–6.

[42] Mander R, Page M. Midwifery and the LGBT midwife. Midwifery 2012; 28: 9–13.

[43] Jones KM, Pynor RA, Sullivan G, Weerakoon P. A Study of Attitudes toward sexuality issues among health care students in Australia. Journal of Lesbian Studies 2002; 6(3–4): 73–86.

Chapter 9

Breaking Down Taboos Concerning Sexuality among the Elderly

Doroteja Rebec, Igor Karnjuš, Sabina Ličen and
Katarina Babnik

Additional information is available at the end of the chapter

http://dx.doi.org/10.5772/59302

1. Introduction

Sexuality as a human need for belonging and being close with someone, as a need for affiliation and physical pleasure is typical for all ages in the life span development [1]. In regard to human needs sexuality is a goal (the need) and a mean through which individuals satisfy their needs. Sexuality has a significant impact on individual's self-esteem, well-being, and functioning; it includes personal, cultural and social identity, and not just sexual orientation and behaviour [2]. The need for sexuality and intimacy is maintained in old age [3], only modes of sexual expression can be different concerning individual's age. In addition to physical sexual relations elderly can express sexuality through hugging, fondling, kissing, holding hands, touching or physical closeness [3, 4], through demonstrating mutual tenderness, support, and understanding, and through developing a new partnership relationship [5].

There are many factors that positively or negatively affect the expression of sexuality among elderly in nursing homes. Not only age-related changes and diseases [6] but also some psychosocial factor occurs. Skoberne [7] and Ziherl [6] argues, that these factors are widowhood, separations, quality of partnership, self-esteem, health impact on partnership, economic situation and environmental influence. In fact, sometimes is easier to influence on age-related changes and disease than environmental influence which has a significant impact on satisfaction of sexual needs in older age. Moreover, in this case the environmental influence means other people views whether are already so deeply entrenched and changing them can be very time consuming process. Society still perceives older people without sexual needs or incapable of sexual activity. For that reason elderly suppress their sexual needs and start to behave in accordance with these beliefs [7].

Institutional care is important and widespread form of care for the elderly who are no longer able to live independently. The attitude of nursing staff towards sexuality is very different and may vary from positive to negative or permissive and restrictive [8]. This can significantly inhibit the expression of sexuality among the elderly. Room designs which do not provide privacy [9], taking care just for the physical needs, avoid talking about sexuality because of the shame [1, 10, 11], failure to respect residents autonomy or the need to control their behavior [3], and letting families to take decisions instead of them [12] are the aspects which may have a significant impact on sexual or intimacy expression among elderly living in nursing homes. Moreover, nursing staffs day-to-day contact with residents often develops into strong relationships, which also affect the sexual expression of the elderly in nursing homes [13]. Since satisfaction of needs has an important role in individual's satisfaction, happiness, and wellbeing, the study of nursing care professionals' attitudes toward sexuality and sexual needs of elderly is necessary for a comprehensive understanding of the determinants which influences the quality of life among elderly in nursing homes. In the end of the chapter authors present the results of a study of nursing care professionals' attitudes toward sexuality of elderly in nursing homes which was performed on a sample of nursing staff from 5 Slovenian nursing homes. The authors developed a semantic differential scale, encompassing a list of adjectives, through which nursing care professionals described the meaning attached to sexuality of elderly in institutional care.

2. Physiological and psychosocial aspects of sexuality among elderly

Older people continue to have need for maintaining their sexual activity and intimacy [3], they just change the ways of expression of their needs. However, in addition to physical sexuality, elderly express their sexuality also with hugging, caresses, kissing, holding hands, touching or by physical closeness [3, 4] as well as tenderness, partners support and mutual understanding [5]. There are many factors that positively or negatively affect the expression of sexuality among elderly which include not only age-related changes and diseases [6] but also some psychosocial factors.

Over the years, some *physiological* changes occur in aged population that affects their sexual activity. For example, men take longer to get an erection, which can be shorter, and women can perceive physiological changes as a vagina moistening problem. However, Walsh and Berman [14] observed that with age the desire for sexual activity and the possibility of experiencing orgasm do not decrease. Although, in the recent years, studies that describe sexual lives among older women become more frequently, we still trace down some prejudices that with the menopause sexual life is over or that sexuality during menopause is not appropriate [15].

The level of estrogen in women after menopause is declining, but the body still produces enough testosterone to maintain interest in sex [15, 16]. Some women after 60 years may experience that the clitoris is somewhat reduced, but still remains very sensitive [17]. Also, due to dryness and vaginal atrophy women can experience pain during sexual intercourse

http://dx.doi.org/10.5772/59302

(dyspareunia) [16]. Sexual excitement can be reduced or it is weaker, and therefore women require a longer petting to lead her to an orgasm [15]. There also may be some psychological symptoms that accompany menopause. The fact that women in menopause cannot have children any more, for some proves the inevitable aging [14, 18]. Distress in older women is also caused by other factors including urinary incontinence, removal of the uterus and some other chronic diseases [19], although the removal of the uterus usually does not affect sexual satisfaction [16]. However, all this have an impact not only on the sexual functioning, but also on emotional state, self-esteem and consequently interpersonal relationship [20].

Even older men are confronted with some changes that may affect the perception of sexuality and sexual desire, although most of them produce enough testosterone that is sufficient to maintain libido [16]. The most common sexual dysfunction in man is erectile dysfunction and hypogonadism [20]. In fact, erectile dysfunction in man increases with each decade, starting at age 60 [21]. Masters and Johnson [17] found that men aged between 50 and 90 years, usually state that their erection is slow and incomplete, and for its maintenance need more stimulation. In older men the stimulation should be of both, mental and physical nature in contrast to younger men which mostly require only mental stimulation. On the other hand, older men have the ability to have greater control over ejaculation, but the intensity and volume of ejaculate is smaller [22]. Same authors also indicate a shorter orgasms and prolonged interval between each ejaculation. For those aged more than 70 the interval can be extended up to 48 hours [16], but it rarely happens that a sex organ is completely unresponsive [23]. Even some health problems and chronic diseases may affect the sexual performance in older man. Diabetes, vascular disease, fear of heart attack, certain operations (for example prostatic surgery) and some medications (used to treat hypertension, depression, anxiety, cancer etc.) can affect sexual desire or ability to have sexual intercourse [14, 23]. Table 1 presents some of the key changes among elderly man and woman that affect their sexuality and sexual functioning.

Physiological changes in men	Physiological changes in women
• slow excitation	• dryness and vaginal atrophy
• reduced ejaculate volume	• shorter and narrowed vagina
• smaller intensity of ejaculate	• reduced vaginal discharge
• shorter erection	• shorter clitoris
• incomplete erection	
• a longer unresponsive period before re-erection	

Table 1. Physiological changes among elderly [19]

Sexuality among elderly has also some advantages. Master and Johnson [17] have stated that one of the advantages of aging, according to the sexual functioning is that the control of ejaculation in the man aged 50 to 70 is better than in man aged between 20 to 40. In other words, many older people retain the ejaculation longer and therefore the sexual intercourse last longer to orgasm. Furthermore, women are no longer afraid to become pregnant [23] and they no longer need the contraceptives, which can release libido and lead to an increased desire for sexual contact [18].

But in spite of this society still perceives older people without sexual needs or incapable of sexual activity. For that reason elderly suppress their sexual needs and start to behave in accordance with these beliefs [7]. Lindau et al. [24] found, that sexual desire and activity are widespread among elderly man and women; however those aged more than 70 placed less importance on sex than the younger population [25]. The same authors also found that there are some gender differences in attitudes toward sexuality, with the greatest difference being in the older age group (41,2 % of males aged 75 – 85 stated an interest in sex compared with 11,4 % of females of same age) [24]. Other studies also shown that not having sexual partner and having poor health status in the late period of life are associated with decreased sexual activity [26, 27], but this does not necessarily mean that sexuality is not important to older people. In fact, Gott et al. [25] found that only when the barriers to remain sexually active were too great to be overcome then sex assume no importance, regardless of age.

Psychological aspect may be as important as physiological aspect for sexual function because this aspect can impact the ways in which other determinants of sexual function are expressed [28, 29]. For example, emotional and interpersonal motivation mediates the effect of sexual desire which is produced by neuroendocrine mechanisms. In fact, motivation plays an important role regarding personal attitudes about sexuality [28] and in sexual functioning of the person because it may increase the desire for sexuality and affects on sexual inactivity due anxiety, or anger with partner [30]. Psychological problem such as depression also influence sexual function in all age group. Its pharmacological treatment is associated with sexual dysfunctions such as anorgasmia, erectile dysfunction, diminished libido that may persist even after medication use is discontinued [31]. However, sexual dysfunction in depressed older adults is often overlooked and less appropriately treated than in younger population [20]. Moreover, psychological aspect is independently related to sexual function. Self-perception theory argues that individuals make attributions about their own attitudes, feelings, and behaviors by relying on their observations of external behaviors and the circumstances in which those behaviors occur [30]. Self-perception theory can be applied to a situation in which a woman observes that she is receptive to her partner sexual initiations, but she is never the initiator. Consequently, the woman perceives that because she engages in sexual activity only in response to her partner, she has low sexual desire [16]. Also, many women because of self-perception theory and overjustification, experience sex as an obligation rather than as an enjoyable part of the relationship, and they consider themselves sexually inadequate. Low self-esteem or poor body image due to aging is also an important psychological barrier which affects the sexual activity of older adults [17]. Furthermore, many couples in long-term relationship perceive the natural decrease in excitement and passion as a symptom of failed marriage. But in every long-term relationship passion can decline over the time and comfort, security, and partnership step in [28]. In addition, relationship duration may affect sexual frequency. Call et al. [32] found that the habituation to sex occurred as relationship duration increased, resulting in a decline in sexual frequency. However, sexual frequency decline is not synonymous with the decline in sexual satisfaction. Gott and Hinchliff [7] also found, that in older adults age was seen as facilitating cooping when sex become less frequent, or stopped. It seems that for older adults in long-term relationship is normal that sex will become less possible with normal ageing and the cessation of sex is easier to cope.

As mentioning before, sexuality is affected by several aspects which plays a crucial role in sexual functioning among elderly. One of them is also *social* aspect which includes many factors, like gender, race, ethnicity, educational and environmental background, socioeconomic status, financial resource, and religion that affects the sexual activity in older adults [21, 28]. Huffstetler [17] emphasized that internalizing negative attitudes toward sexuality and the lack of available partners are the most important social barriers in older adults. In this context DeLamater and Karraker [30] also stated that for older adults the availability of a partner seems to be an important factor for sexual functioning. Although studies [25] indicate that man population is more sexually active, Lindau et al. [24] found that the difference in overall rates between man and woman is manly explained by the relative shortage of man which is in turn due to disparity in ages between partners. In fact, men tend to be older than their spouses but also there is present higher longevity among woman which in older ages results in a shortage of man in later life period [30]. Therefore, Gott and Hinchliff [25] found that older people who are not in relationship or are widowed plays lesser importance on sex. Relationships factors are important because it is difficult to isolate sexual function out of this context, and the presence or absence of partner affects sexual desire [30]. Most of older people think about sexuality as an important component of close emotional relationship in later life and express no interest in sex outside this context (for example in the form of "one night stands") [25]. Laumann et al. [33] found in their analysis of the Global Study of Sexual Attitude and Behaviors that sexual satisfaction and relationship satisfaction are highly related in older adults, which means that for aged population sex in companionate relationship also express the quality of the relationship. The same authors [33] also found that men reported higher levels of subjective sexual wellbeing regardless of sociocultural context than did woman. Older men are less likely than older woman to state that they do not enjoy in sex [21]. Besides, in the society still persist some double standards between the genders which can be explained by the cultural myth that men have greater sexual needs. In fact, when man engage in sexual activity outside the bounds of marriage it is much more acceptable, and it is often viewed as necessary for remaining healthy, whereas women adulterers are often viewed as selfish or whorish [17]. But most older adults still think that sexuality is something that is not appropriate in adult life. In fact, older adults' may internalize the stereotype of sex in older age being wrong [20]. One Finnish study [34] showed that although many older adults have an active sex life, more than half were of the opinion that sexually active life in older age is somehow inappropriate. Also cultural experiences and cohort effects are important factor in sexual expression. The oldest individuals borne before the sexual revolution are now 65 years or more and their sexual attitude differs from the generations born before them. So called "Baby Boom" generation in the period of adolescence enjoyed the sexual expression and many of them enjoy it even today [30]. Researcher [35] found a significant correlation between sexual power among the youth, middle and older man population which means that "Casanova" in the young age remains "Casanova" in the later period of life. Another important sociocultural aspect is the religion which has also a great impact on individual's attitude toward sexuality, especially among older adults in western societies [17]. During the middle Ages, the European church decreed that sexual intercourse was solely for the purposes of procreation. In fact, older individuals who have more conservative religious beliefs are looking at the sexual intercourse and masturbation in the postmenopausal period as something with negative connotation; because this kind of sexual activity does not include the possibility of procreation they perceive it as a sin [17]. Others social aspects can also have a great influence on the sexual activity in older people, like socioeconomic status (individuals with lower socioeconomic status are more sexually active) or ethnicity (among older adults, African Americans are more sexually active than Caucasians) [17] as well as environmental restrictions, in case of communal living environment (e.g. nursing homes), where the lack of privacy may force some residents to express their sexuality in semiprivate or public places [21].

3. Nursing care professionals' attitudes towards sexuality among elderly in nursing homes

3.1. Stereotypes about sexuality in elderly

Sexuality is an intrinsic part of human being, but evidence still suggests that in elderly this area of life is often overlooked, particularly in long-term care settings [36]. Madsen [37] argue that society is a barometer for how majority feels about a certain topic such as sexuality in later life, so the societal views can be used as a guide for where changes may be needed or should be done. We may assume that society indicates, but at the same time determines the point of view about sexuality in later life. Sexuality is still stereotypically seen as something normal, desired, acceptable and meaningful when it comes to young people, but in older sexuality is perceived as unnecessary, pointless, embarrassing and even disturbing [13, 37-39]. Such a stereotypical viewing arises from reflecting on the elderly as unattractive, asexual and unable to get involved into intimate and sexual relationships [7] and leads to the misconception and wrong conclusion that elderly have no such needs.

3.2. Impact of stereotypes about sexuality in elderly on a perception of elderly, their relatives and nursing staff

Stereotypes about sexuality in elderly (mentioned above) may have several effects. They may affect the perception of older people themselves but also the perception of others that coexist with the elderly in the same environment (e.g. caregivers, relatives). How the elderly in nursing homes feel about their own sexuality is similar to older adults in general: interest in sex does not necessarily diminish with admission to a nursing home but engagement in sexual behavior often does [36]. According to Villar et al. [39] a large proportion of elderly pushed the sexuality aside and do not think about it anymore. Social taboos associated with sexuality in older age predominate even because many older people are still caught between their own need for intimacy but also the need to fulfill societal expectation [36]. Today's elderly still belong to the

http://dx.doi.org/10.5772/59302

generations that were raised up in a restrictive and repressive way, but also under the influence of religion and religious education [39]. These generations think about sex as a topic that should be hidden and shall not be spoken about, because it only makes sense in terms of procreation, otherwise it can be socially and morally inappropriate in old age. This contributes to the invisibility of sexuality in old age in general. Sexual needs of older people are often ignored and overlooked by society in general and particularly in long-term care settings so the nursing care professionals have difficulties distinguishing between appropriate and inappropriate sexual expression and behavior by elderly in nursing homes [36].

Such a stereotypical point of view has an impact on the perception and consequently on attitudes of those who live nearby elderly (e.g. relatives caring for old parents in domestic environment) or are professionally involved with elderly (e.g. nursing care professionals in institutional care units or residential care facilities). Villar et al. [39] argue that a group pressure which partly derived from elderly and partly from relatives and nursing care professionals on the other side is an important factor of inhibiting sexual interest and expression. That pressure contribute to controlling behavior of elderly – the importance of what other people think about someone's sexual behavior might cause in elderly feelings of being judged and ashamed or even guilty. Roach [9] in Mahieu [13] state that perception of nursing care professionals and the ethos in the organization where they work are the main factor influencing nursing staff' attitudes toward older adults' sexuality in institutional care settings. Roach [9] points out that nursing staff perceptions and responses to residents' sexual behavior were influenced by their own level of comfort related to sexual issues as well as organizational ethos. Furthermore, nursing staff attitudes influence vice versa their own perceptions about sexual expression of elderly and the extent to which the expression is considered to be problematic or not [36]. At this point it should be noted a reverse impact of nursing care professionals' attitudes and the organizational ethos not just on well-being and self-image of residents but also vice versa on nursing staff themselves. If nurses often feel embarrassed and helpless about resident's sexual behavior (especially when uninhibited sexual behavior occurs in elderly with dementia) it might be detrimental for their self-image and causes negative experiences among them [13]. As stated previously, nursing staff experiences are affected by their own level of comfort related to sexual issues and the organizational ethos, but this in turn has an impact on staff' emotional and behavioral responses to the resident' sexuality [36]. We could conclude that there is a complex and reciprocal interaction between experience, perception and attitudes of nursing care professionals on the one side, then organizational culture of nursing home on the other side, but also the perception of what is wright and what is considered to be wrong among residents and their relatives. All these factors should be considered when exploring the effects on sexual expression among old people living in nursing homes.

3.3. Impact of institutional environment

Due to a complex interaction of various factors (mentioned above) the institutional care settings, where elderly could live for many years, represent an important and challenging area if we want to respect a right of elderly to express their sexual needs [13, 39]. Expression of sexual needs among elderly in nursing homes could be also a very sensitive subject for many nursing care professionals and family members due to a variety of ethical issues and concerns, especially when dementia residents are involved because it might easily be perceived as a behavioral problem rather than the expression of human need to love and intimacy [38]. Skoberne [7] and Ziherl [6] argues that environmental factors which could have a significant impact on sexual expression among institutionalized elderly, are sometimes much more difficult to cope and change than other factors (e.g. age-related changes or diseases). According to their experience the people's view might be so deeply embedded and persistent that changing it can be a very long process.

According to Madsen [37], the institutional environment is for the elderly in many ways very restrictive. Nursing home could be an environment which may directly or indirectly limit elderly or even makes them unable to establish and maintain intimate relationships with another person. Causes of such limiting effect are many, but at the end they all lead to lack of privacy which is essential in intimate relationship. The opportunities for institutionalized old people to express their sexual needs are determined both by architectural features and institutional policy. The most common barriers to sexual expression of elderly in nursing homes derived from facility design and how the work processes are performed (institution policy, organizational protocols, rules, guidelines, instructions etc.) The result is an organized, structured and in some way directed daily life of residents. All the facts shown in Table 2 are recognized as important elements in restricting old people rights for privacy by various authors [10, 37, 39, 40].

It seems that the main causes which are indicating a denial of sexuality among elderly by nursing care professionals are the lack of privacy and restriction of the individual person in different ways, both pointing to negative nursing staff attitudes. Personal beliefs, embarrassment and thinking that sexual expression may potentially have a disruptive effect on life in nursing homes seemed to be reasons why sexual expression of elderly is sometimes considered unacceptable [36]. Barriers mentioned in a Table 2 could be indirect indicators of negative attitudes toward sexuality in elderly. It is not only nursing staff members who may act in a negative way toward sexual expression of elderly but also managers of the institution. They may have an even greater impact on how the sexuality of elderly is accepted because of providing working conditions in the institution. As Table 2 shows one could think about listed barriers that major responsibility for attitudes toward sexuality in elderly lies on factors which seem to be dependent just on a nursing home policy and how the working processes must be carried out. But if you think about listed barriers more accurately, we can conclude that the listed causes are, after all, a result of individual's attitudes that subsequently influence the institutional culture and policies about sexual behavior in nursing homes. From that point of view the listed factors are indirect indicators of attitudes toward discussed topic, but have a direct impact on how nursing staff deals with sexual desires and needs for intimacy of residents in nursing homes.

http://dx.doi.org/10.5772/59302

Facility design
• semi-private rooms (even more than two residents together in the same room)
• absence of individual rooms or bathrooms
• common living areas for residents
• facility designed as a hospital with quick access to residents and living areas
Institution policy, organizational protocols and working procedures
• unlocked-door policy and removal of keys by staff because of safety and surveillance (residents are forced to hide and lock in bathroom for some privacy)
• absence of not disturbing signs
• lack of roommate choice
• separation from partner
• enforced selection of the company for spending most of day time in common dining room and other places for socializing
• structured daily life, standardized schedules and emphasizing communal activities (rather than resident decides how to spent their free time)
• structured ways how to do stuff by self in nursing home facilities - predetermined way to do something or perform something (e.g. when and how to do a bath or a personal hygiene)
• restrictive clothing (in a way to restrict an access to the body or parts of the body)
• constant presence of nursing staff and attendants
• supervision of daily activities and relationships of elderly (by nursing staff and attendants)
• day and night checks by nursing staff
• regulation requiring residents to remain indoors between specified hours (especially at evening or at night)
• sharing the personal data of residents among nursing staff (data may become the subject of discussions, gossip, mocking and laughing or other ways for the inappropriate use of humor as a means of social control)
• informing relatives and adapting things to their expectations to avoid problems
• making decisions in consent of relatives but without resident permission or regardless of her / him wishes
• using a medical model approach to care where staff assume the role of decision-maker and establish routines that facilitate working processes without disruption, but also with little or none consideration about what residents' needs about sexual expression are

Table 2. Barriers to residents' sexual expression in nursing homes [10, 37, 39, 40]

At this point we must also consider the aspect of residents' safety. According to Madsen [37] the reason that most current policies and procedures are restrictive about sexual expression of elderly is that of ensuring safety. This seems to be especially important when it is about to protect a cognitive or physically impaired residents which may not be able to make decisions about any sexual activities. In addition there is a possibility of sexual abuse or exploitation by other resident, even partner. This is supported also by Mahieu et al. [38] who claim that principle of respecting the autonomy is most mentioned factor in assessing the permissibility for sexual behavior in institutionalized elderly persons, but only when elderly person is still capable to make decisions. If elderly suffer from mental and/or physical deterioration their need and desire for sexual fulfillment and intimacy is being denied – resident is seen only as a patient [38] in which we think that the physical needs must be fulfilled first and that only physical needs should be met. This (medical) point of view does not support a holistic approach in nursing care of elderly. It shows that nursing staff is thinking about sexuality in elderly as unimportant and useless and consequently would not promote this area of life of the elderly. Even more, caregivers think that nothing bad happens if this area remains neglected [1, 11]. This avoidance is consistent with the findings of Villar et al. [39] that under the pretext of "ensuring safety" lays tendency to avoid problems regarding sexual behavior and to satisfy expectations of relatives.

3.4. Nursing care professionals' attitudes towards sexuality among institutionalized elderly

It is already clear that the sexuality among institutionalized elderly is a delicate topic from many aspects. Therefore, at the beginning we must always ask, what is our position on the topic – and therefore what is the point of view about sexuality in nursing homes among employees. In nursing homes residents and staff are in constant contact so they both develop strong interpersonal relationships which affect sexual expression in elderly [13]. In the field of exploration the nursing care professionals' attitudes towards sexuality among the elderly in nursing homes suggest a certain discrepancy between different authors. Bouman et al. [8] have found both positive and negative staff attitudes. More likely to have a positive attitude are employees with higher educational level, higher socio-economic status and many years of work experience. But on the other side, a predictive of negative attitude to late life sexuality are younger staff, less than five years experiences of working in nursing home, working with high dependent residents and also in the case of strong religious beliefs [41]. On the other hand, Madsen [37] finds no relationship between staff age, years of working experience and attitudes, although it considers that this could be expected because of similar life-stage and consequently experiencing to be peers by age. Nevertheless Mahieu et al. [13] draw attention to the potential impact of methodological approaches in research-studies with a quantitative approach show more positive attitudes and those with qualitative approach more negative attitudes. On their opinion the negative climate and the lack of privacy is typical for a nursing home environment, but in spite of this the methodological approach is the factor that need to be considered as a possible cause for discrepancy in the results. In this context Bouman et al. [41] point out the inconsistency in attitude-behavior relationship as the important phenomenon that must be kept in mind when we talk about discrepancy in results. Elias and Ryan [36] emphasize that research about sexuality in elderly is not so much focused on late life sexuality as well, but rather in sexuality and dementia because of concerns and ethical dilemma nursing staff is faced with.

Nevertheless, many authors [13, 37, 38] are uniform in the claim that nursing care professionals still have a rather negative attitudes toward sexual behavior of elderly in institutional care settings, especially in western cultures where ageism and stereotypes are still prevailing. Particularly it is the case in situations where nursing staff experience difficulties in distinguishing between healthy and unhealthy sexual behavior, like in elderly with dementia [13, 37]. The sexual interest of elderly might be perceived as a behavioral problem rather than an expression of basic human needs [38], so the care is focusing on preventing and solving problems emerging from unwanted and unknown sexual behavior rather than the provision of holistic care to elderly, especially in those with dementia [36].

4. A pilot study of nursing care professionals attitudes toward sexuality among institutionalized elderly: Nursing home facilities

4.1. Problem statement

Limited numbers of studies assess attitudes toward sexuality among elderly in nursing care homes [36]. Sexuality of elderly in nursing homes is determined by complex relations between several variables, pertaining to the individual, institution, social milieu and societal culture. The question of how nursing care professionals evaluate sexuality among elderly in the nursing home facilities and which underlying meaning they assign to sexuality among residents of nursing homes can have an important impact especially on institutional practices and policies related to sexual intimacy of the elderly. With the aim to assess nursing care professionals' attitudes toward sexuality of elderly in nursing homes, we performed a pilot study on a sample of Slovenian nursing homes workers. The study had two goals: i) to develop an instrument to assess nursing care workers attitudes toward sexuality among institutionalized elderly and to ii) determine how nurses that work in nursing home facilities evaluate the expression of sexuality among residents of nursing homes.

The instrument for measuring attitudes toward sexuality among institutionalized elderly scale was developed as a semantic differential scale. A semantic differential technique [42, 43] is a multi-item measure used to obtain a relative direct indication of attitude [44] in measuring meaning of objects and concepts. Although a review of methodological research on semantic differential [45] show its limitations, semantic differential is a technique widely utilized in studies examining attitudes and stereotypes toward different objects and concepts, especially in relation to age [46-48] and questions that incorporate stronger affective component, such as the women's attitudes toward menopause [49]. Ajzen [50] notes that semantic differential has been in previous studies employed as a measure of affect toward the object and also as a measure of cognition, and concludes that "it is thus possible, by carefully selecting appropriate scales, to use the semantic differential to assess and attitude's cognitive or affective component." [50]. Since previous studies [37] show that sexual behavior of elderly in institutional care settings is connected with rather negative reactions of nursing staff and with stereotypes toward older people, we can expect a stronger affective component of nursing staff attitudes toward perceived sexuality among elderly in nursing care facilities. The differential scale technique is therefore a good approach for the development of a scale that measures evaluations and reactions of nursing care professionals toward sexuality of elderly. In the next section we present the procedure of the development of the attitudes toward sexuality among institutionalized elderly scale.

4.2. Method

4.2.1. Instrument: Scale development and scale description

The attitude toward sexuality among institutionalized elderly scale development process included three stages: i) the identification of adjectives through which nursing care professionals describe and evaluate perceived expressions of intimate relations between elderly in nursing homes, ii) the formation of a list of adjectives that represent evaluations of perceived intimate relations between elderly in nursing homes, and iii) the formation of a list of bipolar sets of adjectives that describe attributes and behavioural characteristics of intimate relations between institutionalized elderly from the perspective of nursing care professionals.

The adjectives through which nursing care professionals describe and evaluate perceived expressions of intimate relations between elderly in nursing homes were identified through a focus group with students, enrolled in the second cycle bologna study programme of nursing care. In the focus group 15 students participated, the majority of them already employed and with experience in nursing practice, two of them also in nursing home facilities. Two questions were discussed with focus group members: i) how do you, as a nursing care professional, evaluate different forms of expression of intimacy and sexuality between elderly in nursing home facilities, ii) is there any discrepancy between your evaluations as a person and as a nursing care professional – if yes; why such differences in evaluations exists? Examples of evaluations of the theme that have emerged during the focus group are: "Well, it is god for their health, although sometimes disturbing for us, as health care workers", "It's embarrassing."…"It can be perceived aggressive or better determinant… but on the other hand it is their intimacy… until it is spontaneous or honest...". "It's not easy; we know that this is something ordinary, spontaneous, frequent." From responses of focus group interview 51 adjectives through which nurses evaluate perceived sexuality and intimacy of elderly in nursing home facilities were identified. From the list, synonyms and similar adjectives were excluded, resulting in a list of 31 adjectives.

In the second step the list of 31 adjectives was discussed with the second group of 21 nursing care students, enrolled in the second cycle bologna study programme of nursing care. Also the second group of students included participants with experience in nursing care practice, also in nursing home and other forms of health care facilities for older people. The discussion was directed toward the validation of identified adjectives (comparison with personal experience) and overall evaluation of the list of adjectives. In the second step a list of 26 adjectives was identified.

From the final list of 26 adjectives we formulated a list of bipolar sets of adjectives (26 items) that describe evaluations intimate relations between institutionalized elderly (older than 75 years) from the perspective of nursing care professionals. The adjectives incorporate the evaluations of behavioural characteristics of the object of evaluations (*strong, frequent, intensive, spontaneous*) and the attributes assigned to the object from the perspective of nursing care professionals that perceive intimate relations (*tolerant, liberal, disrupting, acceptable*). The instruction for respondents was developed in accordance to the Rosencranz and McNevin's [48] formulation, adapted to the object of evaluations. Each of the 30 scales was scored from 1 to 7, for example: Healthy 1-2-3-4-5-6-7 Un-healthy; Frequent 1-2-3-4-5-6-7 Seldom; Intimate 1-2-3-4-5-6-7 Public.

4.3. Sample

In the pilot study 106 nursing care professionals participated, employed in 5 different nursing homes in Slovenia. In the sample 88 % nursing care professionals were female. The majority of participants were aged between 35 and 50 years (56 %). Participants with finished at least secondary nursing education (88 %) are working in nursing homes as nurse assistants; participants that have finished at least a bachelor nursing study programmes (12 %) are working as registered nurses.

4.4. Data analysis

In the pilot study we performed the reliability and dimensional structure analysis (varimax and oblimin exploratory factor analysis) of the attitudes toward intimate relations between institutionalized elderly scale and calculated the descriptive statistics of the 26 items.

4.5. Results

We performed exploratory factor analysis (principal component) with varimax and oblimin rotation. The factor analysis produced two factors (Table 3) that explain 46,7 % of variance in evaluations of intimate relations between institutionalized elderly. Correlation between factors is 0,26. During the factor analysis two adjectives were excluded from the scale: *friendly* and *aggressive*. Both loaded strongly on separate factors and lowered the level of internal consistency of the scale. The final version of the scale (presented in the Table 3), with 23 items and two-dimension structure has appropriate level of internal consistency (Chronbach's alpha=0,91). The first factor (34,8 % of explained variance) includes adjectives, such as: *safe, healthy, acceptable, spontaneous, pleasant, ordinary*. The second factor (11,9 % of explained variance) includes adjectives, such as: *exciting, intensive, active, frequently*. In accordance with basic three dimensional structure of attitudes – evaluation, potency, activity [50], confirmed also in studies utilising semantic differential scale as a measure of attitudes [45], the first factor obtained in our study incorporates mainly the evaluation dimension of attitudes structure, and the second factor incorporates the activity and the potency dimension. From a more detailed analysis of the adjectives indicating both factors, it is also evident, that the first factor incorporates adjectives that mainly describe the pleasant–unpleasant dimension of reactions toward the studied concept, and the adjectives describing the second dimension includes adjectives that indicate the arousal-activation reactions. The pleasant-unpleasant and the arousal-activation have been consistently found as dimensions describing the emotional terms or the affective component of attitudes [50]. The adjectives included in the attitudes toward intimate relations between institutionalized elderly scale represent evaluations strongly connected to affective responses toward the studied attitudinal object.

Table 3 also shows the descriptive statistics for the scales; the mean values for the items range from M=3,21 (bipolar adjective: *intimate-public*) to M=4,66 (bipolar adjective: *frequently-rarely*); with standard deviations from SD=1,45 (adjective: *beneficial-detrimental*) to SD=1,74 (adjective: *honest-dishonest*). Ratings of bipolar sets of adjectives show neither extremely positive and neither extremely negative, but rather moderately positive evaluations.

	Descriptive statistics				Components	
Adjectives	**Min**	**Max**	**Mean**	**Std. Deviation**	**Evaluation**	**Activity/ potency**
Safe	1,00	7,00	3,42	1,67	0,42	
Acceptable	1,00	7,00	3,94	1,45	0,42	
Healthy	1,00	7,00	3,28	1,56	0,51	
Ordinary	1,00	7,00	3,65	1,61	0,51	
Liberal	1,00	7,00	3,90	1,62	0,58	
Disrupting	1,00	7,00	3,62	1,50	0,58	
Beneficial	1,00	7,00	3,27	1,45	0,63	
Pleasant	1,00	7,00	3,45	1,58	0,64	
Faithful	1,00	7,00	3,54	1,53	0,65	
Embarrassing	1,00	7,00	4,43	1,73	0,65	
Honest	1,00	7,00	3,98	1,74	0,69	
Satisfying	1,00	7,00	3,67	1,56	0,70	
Tolerant	1,00	7,00	3,51	1,59	0,73	
Intimate	1,00	7,00	3,21	1,59	0,73	
Relaxing	1,00	7,00	3,65	1,64	0,74	
Spontaneous	1,00	7,00	3,35	1,54	0,76	
Determined	1,00	7,00	3,94	1,45		0,48
Painful	1,00	7,00	3,73	1,51		0,60
Strong	1,00	7,00	4,07	1,50		0,61
Exciting	1,00	7,00	3,83	1,56		0,62
Active	1,00	7,00	4,33	1,54		0,73
Frequently	1,00	7,00	4,66	1,58		0,73
Intensive	1,00	7,00	4,26	1,46		0,81

Table 3. Dimensional structure and descriptive statistics of attitude toward sexuality among institutionalized elderly scale

5. Discussion and conclusions

The pilot study of attitudes toward intimate relations between institutionalized elderly scale had two goals: i) to develop an instrument to assess nursing care professionals attitudes toward sexuality among institutionalized elderly and to ii) determine how nurses that work in nursing home facilities evaluate the expression of sexuality among residents of nursing homes. Already during the process of the scale development, especially during the focus groups with nursing care students, the beliefs, behavioral and affective reactions toward the theme (sexuality toward elderly in institutional care) were evoked. For participants of the focus group the theme was embarrassing and needed some time to feel comfortable in their expressions. The dichotomy of the question "what it is right" and "how I feel about that" was clearly expressed in participants comments: "I know, it is something ordinary, it is normal and many times for them a pleasant experience that enhance the quality of their life, but still, I do not feel relaxed, I am embarrassed when I encounter such situations or when they want to discuss about sexuality and intimacy… Probably it is so because we are talking about sexuality, the age of people involved… also the fact that people live in institutions, where thinks must be under "control" all the time." Similar notion of self-justification in avoiding problems and interactions in relation to sexual behavior can be found in Villar et al. [39]. "Having the control over the situation" is a form of similar self-justification as to "ensure safety" [39]. Self-justification is in this case needed as a mean to avoid taboos and social presssures related to them.

The factor analysis of the attitudes toward intimate relations between institutionalized elderly scale suggests that nursing staff attitudes toward sexuality and intimate relations of institutionalized elderly have a strong affective component. Exploring nursing staff attitudes towards sexuality among elderly in nursing homes suggests that this is still a taboo issue. The qualitative phase of the scale development process offers deeper understanding of the evaluations of the theme, more than the assessed evaluations. Therefore in further studies of attitudes toward elderly in institutionalized settings, a mixed method approach is advised. The attitudes toward intimate relations between institutionalized elderly scale needs further studies on its reliability and validity, as well as additional validation of the adjectives included in the scale.

Sexuality of elderly in nursing homes is a complex societal phenomenon with multiple causes arising from different groups of people for a given society coexisting with old people. In a first place it is about attitudes that elderly might have towards their own sexuality. Here we must also take into account their desires and ability to fulfill sexual needs if there are any. A second important factor are relatives with their personal views on sexual life in general what may have a great impact in determining what should be or should be not the sexual lives of their parents living in nursing home. Finally we must consider how life in the institution itself might influence the sexual expression of elderly. Although it seems that the impact on sexuality among elderly depends especially upon the policy of nursing home and work processes, it is basically always influenced by attitudes of the individual. Nursing home policy and staff attitudes seem to be in vice versa relationship. Those attitudes make positive or negative effects on the nursing homes policy about sexual expression in late life, but also a vice versa effect on individuals (nursing staff and residents in nursing homes). To break this vicious circle we have to take into account that only education is not enough. Nursing staff must get also a concrete practical experience working with the elderly. This will allow them to know, recognize and understand, without any judgment, the area of sexuality in institutionalized elderly. Willing to know, understand and accept is a starting point in implementing a more permissive attitude to the sexuality among elderly which can be subsequently resulting in practice through restructured nursing home policies and ways of addressing the elderly when it is to ensure and facilitate their need, desire and rights for close, intimate relationships. A balance between rights of elderly to fulfill their sexual needs and ensuring them safety, on the other hand is a very important and challenging aspect for restructuring nursing home policies in a way that this area of late life would be respected as it must be. This is necessarily associated with cultural and even religion characteristics of society, but also with capability of recognizing the need for more knowledge and tolerance regarding sexual expression in elderly. If we point out that sexuality is an important area of human's life, then is not difficult to recognize the importance of training from an early age in a sense of instilling tolerance and understanding sexuality in different stages of life.

Author details

Doroteja Rebec*, Igor Karnjuš, Sabina Ličen and Katarina Babnik

*Address all correspondence to: doroteja.rebec@fvz.upr.si

University of Primorska, Faculty of Health Sciences, Izola, Slovenija

References

[1] Kautz DD, Upadhyaya RC. Appreciating diversity and enhancing intimacy. In: Mauk KL, editor. Gerontological nursing – competencies for care. Sudbury, Massachusetts: Jones & Bartlett Learning; 2010. p602-625.

[2] Callan MR. Providing aged care services for the gay and lesbian community. Australian nursing journal (July 1993). 2006;14(4) 20.

[3] Bauer M, Nay R, McAuliffe L. Catering to Love, Sex and Intimacy in Residential Aged Care: What Information is Provided to Consumers? Sex Disabil. 2009;27(1) 3-9.

[4] Ginsberg TB, Pomerantz SC, Kramer-Feeley V. Sexuality in older adults: behaviours and preferences. Age and ageing. 2005;34(5) 475-480.

[5] Feldkamp JK. Navigating the Uncertain Legal Waters of Resident Sexuality. Nursing Homes: Long Term Care Management. 2003;52(2) 62.

[6] Ziherl S. Starost in spolnost. In: F Kresal, editor. 1 znanstveni simpozij fizioterapevtov Slovenije. Gerontologija-izzivi in priložnosti v fizioterapiji. Radenci: Zbornica fizioterapevtov Slovenije; 2011. p276-281.

[7] Skoberne M. Spolnost in spolno zdravje-Spolno zdravje, 2. del. Obzor Zdr N. 2004;38(1) 117-127.

[8] Bouman WP, Arcelus J, Benbow SM. Nottingham study of sexuality & ageing (NoSSA I). Attitudes regarding sexuality and older people: a review of the literature. Sexual & Relationship Therapy. 2006;21(2) 149-161.

[9] Roach SM. Sexual behaviour of nursing home residents: staff perceptions and responses. Journal of Advanced Nursing. 2004;48(4) 371-379.

[10] Bauer M, Geront M. The Use of Humor in Addressing the Sexuality of Elderly Nursing Home Residents. Sexuality & Disability. 1999;17(2) 147.

[11] Scherger K, Harty B. Assessment, diagnosis, and planning. In: Hogstel MO, editor. Gerontology – nursing care of the older adult. Albany, N.Y.: Delmar Cengage Learning; 2001. p237-256.

[12] Hogstel MO. Nursing facilities. In: Hogstel MO, editor. Gerontology – nursing care of the older adult. Albany, N.Y.: Delmar Thomson Learning; 2001. p387-408.

[13] Mahieu L, Van Elssen K, Gastmans C. Nurses' perceptions of sexuality in institutionalized elderly: A literature review. International Journal of Nursing Studies. 2011;48(9) 1140-1154.

[14] Walsh KE, Berman JR. Sexual dysfunction in the older woman: an overview of the current understanding and management. Drugs & aging. 2004;21(10) 655-675.

[15] Ziherl S. Spolnost po menopavzi. Zdrav Vestn. 2008;77(III) 69-71.

[16] Creagan ET. Klinika Mayo o zdravem staranju: odgovori za uspešno tretje življenjsko obdobje. Ljubljana: Educy; 2001.

[17] Huffstetler B. Sexuality in Older Adults: A Deconstructionist Perspective. Adultspan Journal. 2006;5(1) 4-14.

[18] Pečjak V. Psihologija staranja. Bled: Samozaložba; 2007.

[19] Fields WC. Sexuality: Not Just for the Young. In: M Eckman, editor. Lippincott's Nursing Guide to Expert Elder Care. Philadelphia: Wolters Kluwer Health/Lippincott Williams & Wilkins; 2011. p309-333.

[20] Taylor A, MA Gosney. Sexuality in older age: essential considerations for healthcare professionals. Age & Ageing. 2011;40(5) 538-543.

[21] Rheaume C, Mitty E. Sexuality and intimacy in older adults. Geriatric Nursing (New York, NY). 2008;29(5) 342-349.

[22] Jagus CE, Benbow SM. Sexuality in older men with mental health problems. Sexual & Relationship Therapy. 2002;17(3) 271-279.

[23] Hillman JL. Clinical Perspectives on Elderly Sexuality. New Yotk: Kluwer; 2000.

[24] Lindau ST, LP Schumm, EO Laumann, W Levinson, CA O'Muircheartaigh, LJ Waite. A study of sexuality and health among older adults in the United States. The New England Journal of Medicine. 2007;357(8) 762-775.

[25] Gott M, Hinchliff S. How important is sex in later life? The views of older people. Social Science & Medicine. 2003;56(8) 1617.

[26] Matthias RE, Lubben JE, Atchison KA, Schweitzer SO. Sexual activity and satisfaction among very old adults: results from a community-dwelling Medicare population survey. The Gerontologist. 1997;37(1) 6-14.

[27] Deacon S, Minichiello V. Sexuality and older people: Revisiting the assumptions. Educational Gerontology. 1995;21(5) 497.

[28] Kingsberg SA. The impact of aging on sexual function in women and their partners. Archives of Sexual Behavior. 2002;31(5) 431-437.

[29] Bancroft JHJ. Sex and aging. The New England Journal of Medicine. 2007;357(8) 820-822.

[30] DeLamater J, Karraker A. Sexual functioning in older adults. Current Psychiatry Reports. 2009;11(1) 6-11.

[31] Csoka AB, Shipko S. Persistent sexual side effects after SSRI discontinuation. Psychotherapy And Psychosomatics. 2006;75(3) 187-188.

[32] Call V, Sprecher S, Schwartz P. The Incidence and Frequency of Marital Sex in a National Sample. Journal of Marriage & Family. 1995;57(3) 639-652.

[33] Laumann EO, Paik A, Glasser DB, Kang J-H, Wang T, Levinson B, et al. A Cross-National Study of Subjective Sexual Well-Being Among Older Women and Men: Findings From the Global Study of Sexual Attitudes and Behaviors. Archives of Sexual Behavior. 2006;35(2) 145-161.

[34] Paunonen M, Haggman-Laitila A. Sexuality and the satisfaction of sexual needs. A study on the attitudes of aged home-nursing clients. Scandinavian journal of caring sciences. 1990;4(4) 163-168.

[35] Pečjak V. Psihologija tretjega življenjskega obdobja. Ljubljana: Znanstveni inštitut Filozofske fakultete, Univerze v Ljubljani; 1998.

[36] Elias J, Ryan A. A review and commentary on the factors that influence expressions of sexuality by older people in care homes. Journal of Clinical Nursing. 2011;20(11/12) 1668-1676.

[37] Madsen T. Nursing home caregivers' attitudes regarding sexual behavior of nursing home residents: A cross sectional survey. http://sophia.stkate.edu/msw_papers/55 [accessed 13 March 2014].

[38] Mahieu L, Gastmans C. Sexuality in institutionalized elderly persons: a systematic review of argument-based ethics literature. International Psychogeriatrics / IPA. 2012;24(3) 346-357.

[39] Villar F, Celdrán M, Fabà J, Serrat R. Barriers to sexual expression in residential aged care facilities (RACFs): comparison of staff and residents' views. Journal Of Advanced Nursing. 2014;00(0) 000-000.

[40] Bauer M. Their only privacy is between their sheets. Privacy and the sexuality of elderly nursing home residents. Journal Of Gerontological Nursing. 1999;25(8) 37-41.

[41] Bouman WP, Arcelus J, Benbow SM. Nottingham study of sexuality and ageing (NoSSA II). Attitudes of care staff regarding sexuality and residents: A study in residential and nursing homes. Sexual & Relationship Therapy. 2007;22(1) 45-61.

[42] Osgood CE. The nature and measurement of meaning. Psychol Bull. 1952;49(3) 197-237.

[43] Osgood C, Suci G, Tannenbaum P. The measurement of meaning. Urbana, IL: University of Illinois Press; 1957.

[44] Ajzen I. Attitudes, Personality and Behavior. Maidenhead: McGraw-Hill International; 2005.

[45] Heise DR. Some methodological issues in semantic differential research. Psychological Bulletin. 1969;72(6) 406-422.

[46] Gluth S, Ebner NC, Schmiedek F. Attitudes toward Younger and Older Adults: The German Aging Semantic Differential. International Journal of Behavioral Development. 2010;34(2) 147-158.

[47] Intrieri RC, von Eye A, Kelly JA. The Aging Semantic Differential: A confirmatory factor analysis. The Gerontologist. 1995;35(5) 616-621.

[48] Rosencranz HA, McNevin TE. A factor analysis of attitudes toward the aged. The Gerontologist. 1969;9(1) 55-59.

[49] Bowles C. Measure of attitude toward menopause using the semantic differential model. Nursing Research. 1986;35(2) 81-85.

[50] Ajzen I. Attitude structure and behavior. In: P AR, Beckler SJ, Greenwald AG, editors. Attitude structure and function. Hillsdale, NJ: Lawrence Erlbaum; 1989. p241-274.